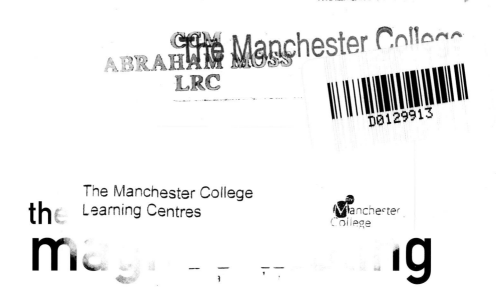

The Manchester College
Learning Centres

the

ma   ng

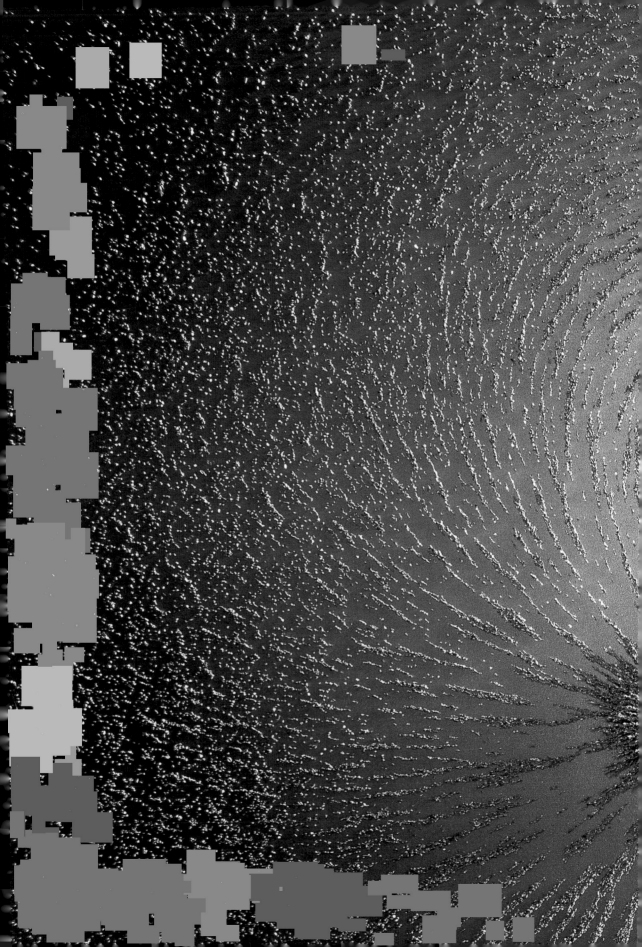

the book of
magnet healing

Roger Coghill

Gaia Books Limited

A GAIA ORIGINAL

Books from Gaia celebrate the vision of Gaia, the self-sustaining living Earth, and seek to help its readers live in greater personal and planetary harmony.

Editors Katherine Pate, Sarah Townsend
Designer Matt Moate
Illustration David Newton and Liz Couldwell
Photography Adrian Swift
Managing Editor Pip Morgan
Production Lyn Kirby
Direction Patrick Nugent

First published in the United Kingdom in 2000 by
Gaia Books Ltd, 66 Charlotte Street, London W1P 1LR
and 20 High Street, Stroud, Gloucestershire GL5 1AZ

ISBN 1-85675-160-0

A catalogue record of this book is available from the British Library.

Printed and bound in Singapore by Kyodo

10 9 8 7 6 5 4 3 2 1

Note on safety
The techniques and treatments in this book are to be used at the reader's sole discretion and risk. Always observe the cautions and consult a doctor if you are in any doubt about a medical condition.

The worldwide availability of this book in the English language has made it necessary to adopt US spellings in certain circumstances, for example, tumor, hemoglobin.

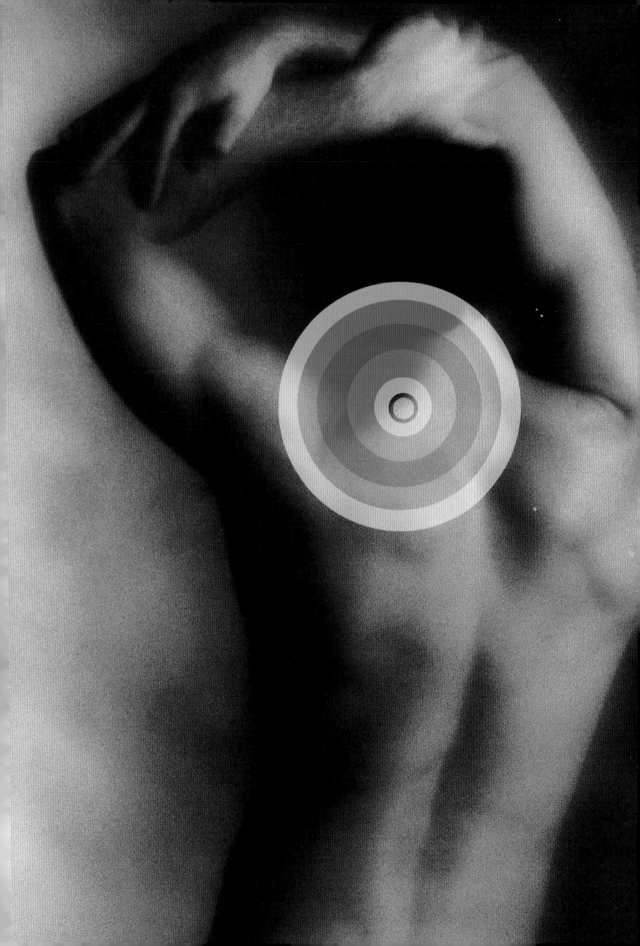

Contents

36 chapter two
your magnetic health

author's preface

The benefits and scope of magnet therapy as a non-invasive and complementary method of healing are still being researched. Each year tens of thousands of people worldwide discover the benefits of this powerful therapy for themselves. Their claims for the success of magnet treatments are both increasing the therapy's popularity and fuelling the demand for further research.

The twentieth century saw remarkable advances in curative medicine, in healthcare, and in the instruments for early diagnosis of illness. Scourges such as smallpox have largely been eradicated around the world; inoculation programmes have restricted some of the previously common infectious diseases such as chickenpox, polio, and mumps. In the industrialized countries, medications such as beta-blockers for heart disease have prolonged the length of life; and at the same time infant mortality rates have fallen dramatically.

In the field of surgery, advance has been nothing short of astounding. A better understanding of immunology has made it possible for organ transplants, hip replacements, implanted cardiac pacemaker technology, and by-pass operations to

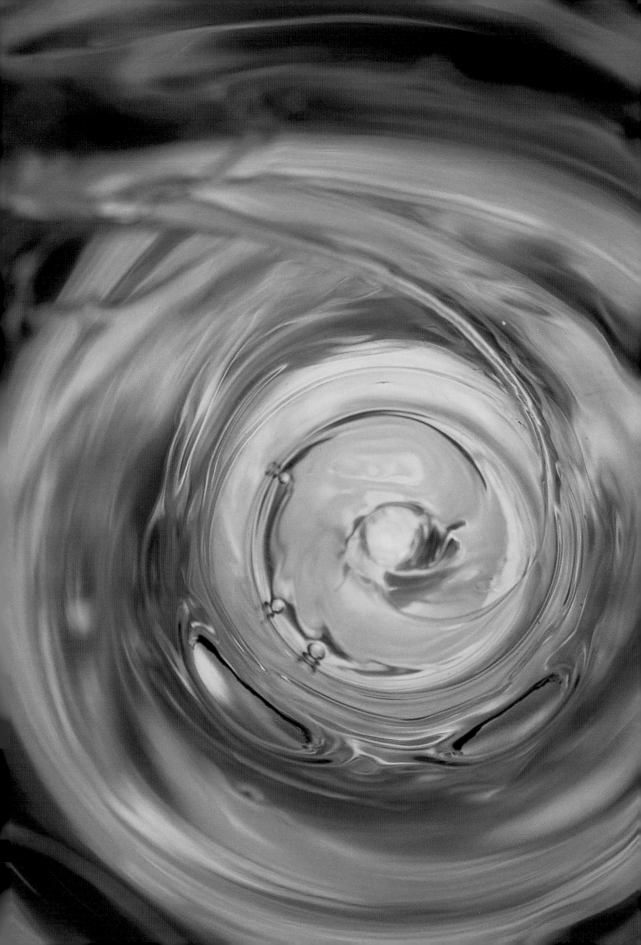

become commonplace. The medical profession has good reason for self-congratulation.

However the picture is not all good. In the western world this past century has also seen a rise in neuro-degenerative diseases such as multiple sclerosis, diseases relating to immune system function, including asthma, and chronic fatigue system, and cancers, including leukemia.

Part of the problem has been the change in lifestyle which has arrived with our new technological world of motor cars, computers, automation, and telecommunications. An ocean of electromagnetic energy from power and telecommunications technologies has flooded the planet in the past fifty years – from high voltage power lines, electricity substations, and radio and cellphone transmitter masts to name but a few. It is becoming increasingly clear that these man-made magnetic and electric fields affect our health and wellbeing. Study after study reports an association between exposure to power, radio, and microwave frequency fields and radiation and an elevated incidence of ill health.

At the beginning of the twentieth century only 10 per cent of workers laboured indoors. Today it is close to 90 per cent. We drive to work, sit all day in an office, drive home again, and on average clock up at least a dozen hours each week watching television. Obesity – due to lack of exercise and a diet rich in sugars, fats, and junk foods – is becoming a major killer, and our sedentary lives are accompanied by lower back pain and a host of other musculoskeletal disorders.

The role of magnet therapy

It is in treating lower back pain and other musculoskeletal problems such as rheumatism and arthritis, that magnet therapy is quietly finding a place. Applying magnets to the affected areas can sometimes deliver spectacular relief in minutes, even to chronic sufferers, and the many anecdotal tales of such effects are borne out by scientific research.

Magnets are also effective in reducing inflammation, whether from burns, sprains, or some toxic agent such as bee or wasp stings. In gout, a painful condition where blood circulation in the foot has been restricted by a build-up of uric acid crystals, magnets help wash the offending crystals away. The Egyptian Queen Cleopatra had never heard of uric acid, but thousands of years ago her physicians knew that static magnets helped relieve gout.

From this basis, research has broadened to investigate magnets' possible use in treating other disorders, and the results list a surprisingly wide array of applications. The use of magnets in medicine has been much more extensive in the Eastern bloc countries and Japan than in the west, where the medical establishment has preferred a pharmaceutical approach.

In 1996 my laboratory organized the First World Congress in Magnetotherapy at London's Royal Society of Medicine, which drew scientists from all over the world. During the proceedings Jiri Jerabek of the Czech Republic presented a paper reviewing magnet healing applications including arthritis, lung disorders, cardiac disorders, neuro-degeneracy, myalgias, and so many other applications that the review was over twenty chapters of close-written technical reports. Other papers included one from Professor Detlavs of Latvia, who recounted his twenty years of clinical experience of healing with magnets. There were also contributions from Japan, where one magnetic products firm is the tenth largest company in that country.

About this book

We have all evolved in the presence of the Earth's magnetic field and this natural magnetism and its effects on us is explored in chapter one. Chapter two illustrates how the advent of artificial electromagnetic fields are detrimental to health and presents practical advice on how to protect yourself from them. The third chapter shows how magnets can assist the natural course of healing in many common conditions. Treatment plans based on the latest research show you where to place the magnets and what results to expect. Finally the resources section provides a comprehensive listing of magnet manufacturers and suppliers, further reading, and magnet institutions worldwide.

R W Coghill

chapter 1
natural magnetism

The seemingly magical force of magnetism has fascinated humankind for centuries. This chapter explores the Earth's natural magnetic field – its rhythms and its variations.

Explanations of the science of magnetism show how magnets affect other materials at an atomic level, and how magnetism is linked with electricity. All living creatures rely on delicate internal electric fields that control the heartbeat, brainwaves, and nerve impulses. These function perfectly in the Earth's magnetic field since they evolved in its presence. But it is easy to see that they can be affected by other magnetic and electric fields. It is this ability of magnets to affect the body and its functions that is the basis of magnet healing.

Since the ancient Chinese learned how to make magnetic compasses, navigators, explorers, and sailors have used the Earth's magnetic field to guide them on journeys across oceans and landscapes. Many animal species also rely on their innate sensitivity to the magnetic field to help them navigate, especially in their long migratory journeys.

The chapter ends with some illustrations of practical uses for magnets – to improve fuel efficiency in car engines, and in pain relief – to indicate their powerful effects and give a fore-taste of the practical magnet healthcare treatments that are presented in chapter three.

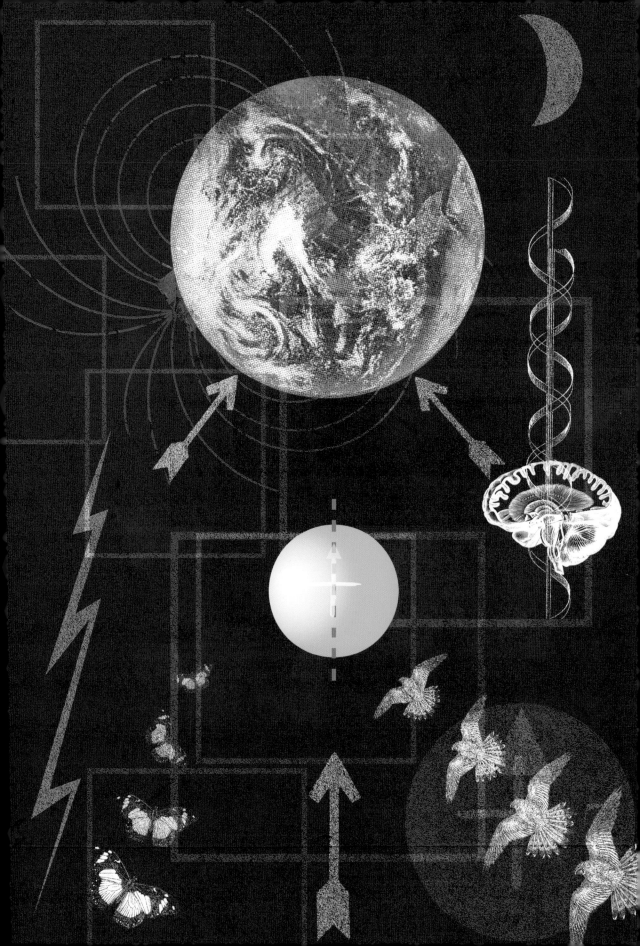

natural magnetism

Many legends surround the mysterious and magical power of magnetism.

Pliny the Elder, a Roman scholar in the first century AD, quoted the legend that Magnes, a Greek shepherd, first discovered natural magnetism in the form of lodestone. His iron staff is said to have been attracted to a lodestone rock so that he was unable to free it. Another legend has it that magnets were discovered first in Magnesia. In classical times there were two cities of this name, in what is now modern Turkey, and there is also a region called Magnesia in Greece, on the mainland facing Chalcidice. These areas were probably all abundant in iron ore. Certainly, in the seventh century BC, the Greek philosopher and mathematician Thales was aware of the magnetic properties of lodestone.

The seemingly magical power of magnetism gave rise to many theories. One that exercised some of the great minds of ancient times was the existence of magnetic islands, which ships could not pass if they had been held together with nails. Ptolemy, the Egyptian astronomer and geographer (AD90–168) believed these islands to lie between Sri Lanka and Malaysia.

Lodestone: the natural magnet

This naturally occurring magnet is an iron-rich ore that has become magnetized through long exposure to the Earth's magnetic field. It retains this magnetism even when it is moved from its original position, and it will attract unmagnetized iron. A small piece of lodestone suspended on a cord will rotate to align itself with the north–south axis of the Earth's magnetic field. It is this ability to point the way that gives it its name, derived from the ancient English word "load" or lead, meaning "to lead the way". It is recorded that St Augustine was greatly surprised by the use of lodestone magnets in Britain on his arrival there in the sixth century AD.

Navigating with magnets

The Chinese first harnessed the power of magnetism to produce the compass. In the Chinese art of Feng Shui calculations were made on a divining board, in the middle of which was the constellation of the Plough as a direction finder. During the Han dynasty (206BC–AD220) the constellation was replaced by a lodestone carved into a spoon shape. It was designed so that it balanced and turned on the underside of the bowl of the spoon. This would align itself with the Earth's magnetic field and was known as "the south-pointing spoon". Eventually the spoon was replaced by other shapes, and by the fifth century AD the Chinese were using needle compasses on land. The next development was the floating water compass, where the piece of lodestone was attached to a splint of wood floating in a bowl of water. Dry suspension compasses followed, where the needle was attached from below, as in modern compasses. These were certainly in use on Chinese ocean-going ships in the eleventh century, a hundred years before they were first used in Europe.

Healing with magnets

As well as their use as navigational aids, magnets have been used in healing through the ages. William Gilbert (1544–1603), physician to Queen Elizabeth I of England, was very interested in the curative properties of lodestone. In his treatise *De Magnete* (On the Magnet) published in 1600 he claimed that a compass had the power to "reconcile husbands to their wives". In this research he dispelled some of the common myths about lodestones: that if pickled in the salt of a sucking fish a lodestone can attract gold, or that onions and garlic can destroy a lodestone's magnetic power. He also disagreed with the practice of taking ground-up lodestone in water for a variety of ailments. This early form of magnet therapy had been prescribed by the Swiss physician and alchemist, Paracelsus (1493–1541).

Other ways that magnets have traditionally been used in many cultures to improve and maintain health are described in chapter three.

the earth as a magnet

We live on a huge magnet and have evolved in its magnetic field.

The Earth's iron-rich crust was magnetized by friction against its molten core long before life first appeared on our planet. We may even owe life itself to the Earth's magnetic field.

The "solar wind" of electromagnetic radiation from the sun distorts the Earth's magnetic field, in the same way as a gust of air distorts a candle flame. Since a moving magnetic field induces an electric current (see page 24) this distortion gives rise to electric currents in the Van Allen Belts, several hundred kilometres above the Earth's surface. Before life evolved there was no protective insulating ozone layer (see right), so these electric currents would have penetrated through the ionosphere to the Earth's core. The resulting bursts of electric energy would have increased the energy available for the chemical reactions likely to give rise to life. Thus magnetism has always been inseparable from life itself, and the fluctuating movements of the Earth's magnetic fields breathe life into our living planet.

There is evidence that the Earth's magnetic field has reversed many times in the past. As magma oozes through cracks in the Earth's crust, its iron atoms align themselves with the Earth's magnetic field, to lie in a north–south direction. As the magma cools it solidifies, creating a snapshot of the Earth's magnetic field at that time. Measurements of such deposits on the Atlantic Ocean bed show that these reversals of the magnetic field have occurred, and have coincided with mass extinctions of fauna. The dinosaurs became extinct at the end of the Cretaceous period when frequent reversals resumed after a long period of inactivity. Similarly, it has been suggested that at the end of the Peruvian period, 225 million years ago, about half of the existing animal species were wiped out. The effect of the reversal of the Earth's magnetic field is probably felt down to the very structure of the molecules of living creatures. The helix structure of DNA has a left-hand

Life on Earth

There was no oxygen before life appeared on the Earth, and hence no ozone layer, since ozone molecules are made up of oxygen atoms, combined in threes. The first life forms to develop were cyanobacteria and then blue-green algae, which create sugar from sunlight by photosynthesis, with oxygen as a by-product. Thus oxygen was available for the development of animal life, and the protective ozone layer began to form.

corkscrew twist, and one theory holds that a change of magnetic field could mean that new DNA would form with a right-hand twist, so old species would die out.

There is no question that the Earth's weak magnetic field can have important biological effects. Some geographical regions have much weaker or stronger fields: the magnetic field is stronger at the poles and weaker at the equator. Also any large deposits of metal ores, or artificial metal structures, tend to concentrate the fields above or below normal levels. The incidence of diseases varies with these differences and phenomena such as slow recovery from illness in slow moving fields, or increased incidences of cancer in fast moving fields, have been noted for decades.

Only recently scientists discovered that even humble mud bacteria are magnetotactic, responding to what seem at first to be exceptionally weak magnetic fields. Some fish, too, can be trained to queue for food when a magnet is swung outside their aquarium. These examples show just how life on our planet is affected by the invisible but powerful force of magnetism.

The rhythms of the Earth

The geomagnetic field is usually described as a static field, but this is not strictly correct. As our great globe revolves on its axis there are tiny changes in the magnetic field strength, which can be detected easily using scientific instruments although the variations are of the order of only 0.2 per cent of the field strength. These fluctuations are due to the structure of the Earth itself. Imagine the Earth as a ball filled with liquid, with another solid ball as its core. As it spins on its axis the liquid inside transmits the spin of the outer shell to the core, making it spin too. But the liquid tends to wobble during the spin, and so the core spins less smoothly and on a slightly different axis to the outer shell. It is this "wobble" effect that causes the observed variations in the Earth's magnetic field. And the different axes of spin of the shell and core create the difference between magnetic north (defined by the north pole of the core) and true north (the north pole of the shell).

The rhythms of the sun

The sun is an uncontrolled nuclear reaction, breaking down atoms into charged particles that are emitted at the speed of light from the sun's surface in solar storms. Observers can see

The natural compass

Our magnetic Earth helps us find our way across featureless oceans. Chinese navigators first discovered that the Earth has a magnetic field and that magnetized needles point to magnetic north. Migrating animals and birds also rely on their sensitivity to this directional cue to find their breeding grounds. But this geomagnetic influence waxes and wanes over long periods, and the direction of magnetic north is slowly changing each year.

occasional black areas on the sun, known as sunspots, which are the result of these gigantic magnetic storms. These sunspots wax and wane in a twenty two-year cycle. In the first eleven years of the cycle (more precisely a mean of 11.135 years) the sunspots are concentrated on one hemisphere of the sun, and in the second eleven years on the other.

Sunspot numbers have been monitored for millennia, and some fifty periods of maximum sunspot activity have been clearly identified between 500BC and AD1600, when telescopes took over the counting. Curiously there have been several "quiet" periods without many sunspots, including a whole period in the seventeenth century (called the Maunder minimum, between 1645 and 1715) when sunspots became comparatively rare and the cycle disappeared for reasons no one has ever explained satisfactorily.

Sunspot influence

In Britain in 1974 Dr Hope-Simpson discovered that all major influenza outbreaks since 1761 have coincided with sunspot maxima, including the 1918 Spanish flu pandemic that killed more than twenty million people worldwide. His finding has been confirmed twice since by astrophysicist Professor Sir Fred Hoyle and his colleagues at Cardiff University, Wales. This remarkable correlation clearly requires an explanation.

The word influenza comes from the Italian word for "influence" because they believed that flu came from some distant agent. Shepherds in the hills of Tuscany would contract the illness on the same day as their friends in the town. On a wider scale, outbreaks of flu often occur in two cities in different continents, so far that case-to-case transmission is impossible, even in these days of high speed travel.

The answer lies with the sun's magnetic fields. At times of sunspot maxima, the solar wind of charged particles is much greater, causing distortions in the Earth's magnetic field. These changes in the field can damage immune competence, leaving us more vulnerable to infection. But the issue is more complicated than that. Strains of flu have their own peculiar characteristics, suggesting that we still do not know all that is involved in flu pandemics.

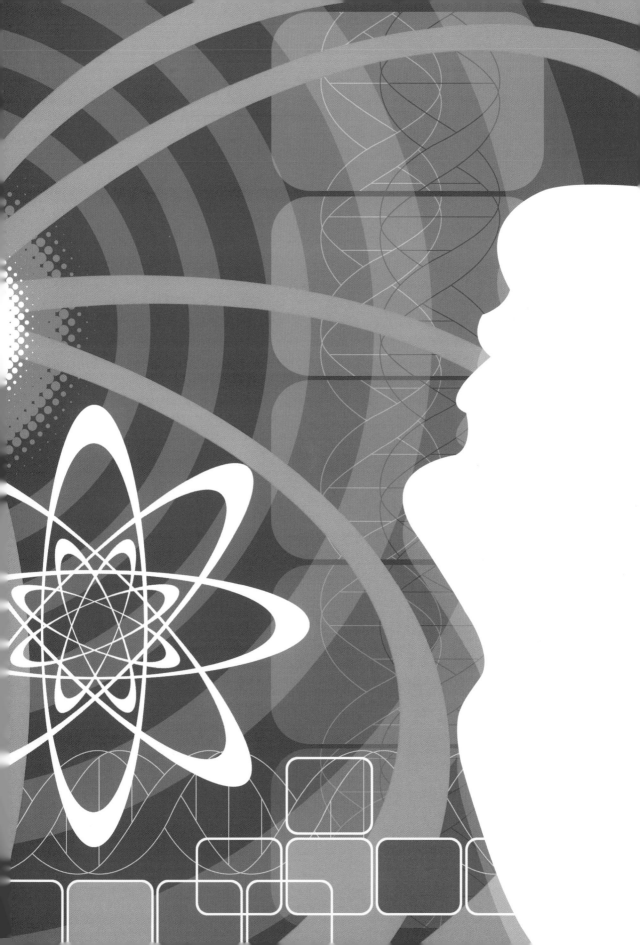

1.

what is a magnet?

The key to magnetism lies in atomic structure.

The structure of an atom

Atoms are made up of three types of subatomic particles: protons, neutrons, and electrons. The protons and neutrons form the nucleus of the atom. The electrons orbit the nucleus in areas of space known as electron shells (1). Protons are positively charged particles, neutrons have no charge, and electrons are negatively charged.

Nature likes balance, even at an atomic level. The charge of an electron is equal and opposite to the charge of a proton, and normally there are an equal number of protons and electrons in an uncharged atom. They are held in the atom by the strong attractive forces between them.

Atoms have up to seven electron shells, and each can hold a certain number of electrons. The inner electron shell holds a maximum of two electrons, the second one eight, and the third a maximum of eighteen.

If the outer electron shell is either full, or contains a group of eight electrons, the atom is unreactive. Atoms with gaps in their outer shells seek to fill them, for example by gaining an electron from another atom.

2.

3.

Within a stable atom or compound the electrons form pairs. In each pair, the electrons spin in opposite directions, or antiparallel, to each other. The iron $Fe(3+)$ atom is an example of an unstable atom. Three electrons are missing from the outer shell, and the unpaired electrons spin haphazardly.

Definition of a magnet

A magnet is a material containing unpaired electrons that all have the same direction of spin, and whose axes of spin are all aligned in the same direction.

An un-magnetized iron bar contains millions of unpaired electrons (2), all spinning in different directions with their axes in different orientations. If the bar is magnetized, all these free electrons spin in the same direction (3), with all their axes in line.

Magnetic field

The field of a magnet is the region around it where objects are affected by its magnetic force. If iron filings are sprinkled around a bar magnet they form a pattern that can be drawn as magnetic field lines (4). The field lines are closer together at the poles of the magnet, where the field is stronger.

4.

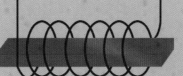

Creating a magnetic field

Electricity's ability to magnetize iron was first discovered by William Gilbert, physician to Queen Elizabeth I, who noticed the magnetizing effect of lightning on iron objects.

Modern magnets are made by placing an iron bar inside a coil of copper wire (5), and passing a strong surge of direct current electricity through the coil. The electricity creates a magnetic field around the coil (see page 00), forcing the unpaired electrons in the iron to line up and spin in the same direction. The direction of the current through the coil determines which is the North and which the South pole.

5.

One way of magnetizing an iron bar is to heat it and leave it to cool lying in a north–south direction. The unpaired electrons all line up in the Earth's magnetic field.

Destroying magnetism

Heating a ferrite magnet to very high temperatures destroys its magnetism, since the electrons are excited by the thermal energy and lose their spin alignment. Hammering a magnet can also have the same effect, by increasing the energy available to the electrons.

6.

7.

How a magnet affects other materials

When a magnet is placed close to a material, its unpaired electrons, all spinning in the same direction, cause any unpaired electrons in the other material to spin too. To picture this, imagine two coins touching each other. If one coin is rotated, the other will begin to rotate, too, but in the opposite direction (6). The direction of rotation holds the two materials together, by magnetic attraction.

The laws of polarity

Opposite forces attract, and like forces repel. With magnets, unlike poles attract (South attracts North and vice versa) and like poles repel. This phenomenon can also be explained by considering the electrons to be spinning like two coins rotating.

If the two coins are rotating in opposite directions (6), i.e. unlike poles, there is attraction. However, if the two coins are rotating in the same direction (7), i.e. like poles, their combined movement will push them apart – repulsion.

modern magnetic materials

Making magnets lighter in weight has created more opportunities for therapeutic use.

Before the time of William Gilbert (see page 15) the only kind of magnet known was the lodestone. But blacksmiths knew that an iron bar could be magnetized by heating it and then beating it with a hammer while it cooled, lying along a north–south axis. Gilbert himself noticed that iron rods left aligned in the Earth's field in that way for twenty years or more became weakly magnetized. He also observed that lightning could magnetize iron.

The traditional horseshoe magnet was developed by bending a straight iron bar magnet into the horseshoe shape. Thus the attractive power of the magnet for an object was effectively doubled by having the two poles side by side. However, since the south and north poles are close together in this type of magnet, they tend to cancel each other out.

The technology for making lightweight, inexpensive, and powerful magnets has improved greatly since those early days, particularly over the last twenty years. And each leap in this development has been accompanied by increased interest in the therapeutic effects of magnets. In the 1700s carbon steel was found to retain its magnetism far better than lodestone or beaten iron. Around the beginning of the twentieth century the first alloy magnets appeared, containing tungsten, cobalt, chromium, or molybdenum. In 1930 iron-based products containing aluminium, nickel, and cobalt were developed, often known as Alnico magnets. All these magnets were metal based and therefore heavy to use.

The first magnets incorporating cobalt and samarium were developed in the 1980s. They were known as rare earth magnets, as they were made from metallic elements from the rare earth group in the periodic table. These magnets were much lighter in weight than any of their predecessors and were developed for industrial uses, such as in electric motors.

Lighter weight magnets
An 8000 gauss Alnico magnet would weigh around 90kg (200lbs). The same strength neodymium magnet would weigh around 20g (0.8oz). A 200 gauss iron magnet weighs around 10g (0.4oz) compared with a 1g (0.04oz) neodymium magnet of the same strength.

However since cobalt and samarium are rare the magnets were also expensive, so in 1983 a variant using iron, boron, and neodymium was developed. These magnets, known as neodymium magnets, are extremely difficult to demagnetize and stay magnetized for decades. They are made by sintering – applying great heat and pressure to powdered metals. This means they are lighter in weight than solid iron or steel magnets, but also brittle, though this disadvantage can be overcome by coating them with chrome or other hard casing metals.

Other mixtures of materials can be magnetic too. In the plastic magnet strips on a refrigerator door the plastic is impregnated with minute magnetic materials, so the strip can be cut to any desired size. Such magnets do not have high field strengths however. Ceramic magnets are also common. These incorporate neodymium and the other rare earth metals and are therefore also capable of high field strengths.

Magnetic field strength

The modern unit of field strength is the tesla (T), named after Nikola Tesla (1856–1943), a Serb who emigrated to New York to work in Thomas Edison's laboratory.

Measuring field strength

The field strength of a magnet is inversely proportional to the square of the distance from it. This means that it falls off very quickly as you move away from the magnet. The strength of the magnetic field of a magnet 4cm (1.7in) away is only one sixteenth its rating at the pole face (on the surface of the magnet); at 8cm (3.4in) it will be one sixty-fourth.

From there he branched out and developed a wide range of the inventions on which our modern society is based, including the ubiquitous fractional horsepower motor. The tesla has largely replaced older units of magnetic field strength, the gauss and the oersted, though the gauss is still in fairly common use, particularly for static magnets used in healing.

Magnets used in healing typically have field strengths in the range 200–2000 gauss. Using the relationship that 1 tesla is the same as 10,000 gauss, it is easy to convert between the two. Since the tesla is a very large unit, therapeutic magnet strengths may be given in thousandths of teslas (milliteslas, mT) or even millionths (microteslas, μT). As an example, 200 gauss is the same as 20mT; 2000 gauss is 200mT.

In magnet healing, stronger is not necessarily better. Some remarkable effects have been achieved with picotesla (10^{-12}T) field strengths, which are exceptionally low. Most reputable suppliers state the strength of their magnets, or at least should be able to tell you if you ask. For therapeutic use it is best to have a selection of magnets of different ratings that can be used in various combinations to apply a range of field strengths.

electricity and magnetism

The forces of electricity and magnetism are linked: one can give rise to the other.

In a now famous experiment first performed unintentionally in 1820 at the Polytechnic Institute in Copenhagen, Hans Christian Oersted (1777–1851), Professor of Physics, discovered that an electric current produces a magnetic field around it.

In a demonstration to his students, Oersted placed a compass needle directly below a wire. When the current through the wire was switched on, the compass needle moved. Further investigation showed that the direction of the current in the wire determined the direction of the magnetic field.

If a wire carrying current is passed through a piece of card sprinkled with iron filings, the filings set into concentric circles around the wire, showing the force lines of the magnetic field. A compass on the card will show the direction of the field. If the direction of current is reversed, the direction of the field also reverses. James Clerk Maxwell, a nineteenth century British mathematical physicist, formulated his "corkscrew rule" to describe the direction of the magnetic field around a wire. If you imagine a corkscrew being screwed along the wire in the direction of the current, then its direction of rotation gives the direction of the magnetic field.

At that time the precise relationship between the two forces of electricity and magnetism was not known. The British scientist Michael Faraday, working in the 1830s, extended Oersted's work on his discovery. He argued that according to Newton's third law (every action has an equal and opposite reaction), the opposite should also be true: a magnetic field should produce an electric current.

Through experiment he showed this to be the case, provided the conducting material or wire cuts the lines of magnetic force. These are the lines that iron filings move into when they are sprinkled around a magnet. Faraday used a bar magnet, which he pushed into a coil of wire. A current was induced in

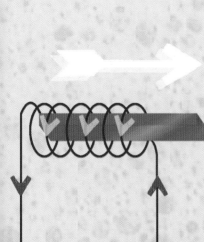

the wire when the magnet was moving, that is, when the wire was cutting through the force lines around the magnet. When the magnet was left stationary inside the coil no current flowed, and when it was pulled out again, current flowed in the opposite direction.

Alternating electric current

The electric current from a battery always flows in the same direction around the circuit and is called a direct current. In contrast, main electricity is alternating current (AC). The direction of the current in the circuit changes many times a second and the frequency of this direction change is measured in hertz (Hz). In the UK main electricity has a frequency of 50Hz; the current switches direction 50 times per second. In the US the frequency is 60Hz; the direction switches 60 times per second.

Since an electric current produces a magnetic field around it, it follows that a wire carrying alternating current produces an alternating magnetic field around it. So moving magnetic fields and electric fields are inevitably linked – each can induce the other.

Static magnetic fields do not have an electric component, since a stationary magnet does not induce a current. We are all comfortable with the static magnetic field of the Earth – we have evolved within it (see page 16). Static magnet fields can also have therapeutic effects, which are described in chapter three. But in the last century we have become exposed to artificial alternating electric fields in our environment as a result of the development of alternating current electricity. The harmful effects that these can have on the body's delicate mechanisms, and how we can protect ourselves from them, are explained in chapter two.

using the geomagnetic field

Nearly all living creatures are sensitive to the Earth's geomagnetic fields.

From bacteria to birds, sensitivity to magnetic fields is built into their anatomy. The mud bacterium *Aquaspirillum magnetotacticum* is an anaerobic bacterium that cannot survive in oxygen. In 1975, Richard Blakemore, a microbiology graduate student at the University of Massachusetts noticed that some of these micro-organisms persistently swam in one direction. A transmission electron microscope photograph revealed a line of tiny black crystals inside the creature's body: magnetosomes (particles of magnetite, an iron-rich compound).

The dip angle of the Earth's magnetic field in the northern hemisphere (see opposite) ensured the magnetosomes tilted the bacterium downward. The flagellations of its tail would then propel it down to the safety of the mud where it lived. Had this species been moved to the southern hemisphere it would have been driven upward to the water's surface and extinction. In 1981 Blakemore found that the species in the southern hemisphere had the reverse polarity. Even when dead the bacteria align with the Earth's magnetic dip angle. There are at least a dozen magnetotactic bacterial varieties which abound in both fresh water and marine environments.

Homing pigeons, migratory salmon, chitons (a variety of marine mollusc), butterflies, and dolphins have since been found to have magnetite inside them. Joe Kirschvink of Caltech, the California Institute of Technology claims to have discovered magnetosomes in the human brain too.

The mystery of migration

Whales migrate across oceans to warm basking and breeding grounds in the Gulf of Mexico. The Mid-Atlantic Ridge, stretching in an S-shape from Iceland to the Antarctic Circle,

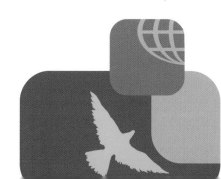

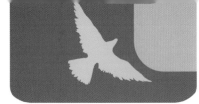

The dip angle

A compass needle aligns itself along the lines of the Earth's magnetic field. In the northern hemisphere the north end of the needle dips toward the Earth's surface. At the equator the dip angle is zero and at the North Pole it is 90 degrees. In the southern hemisphere the situation is reversed.

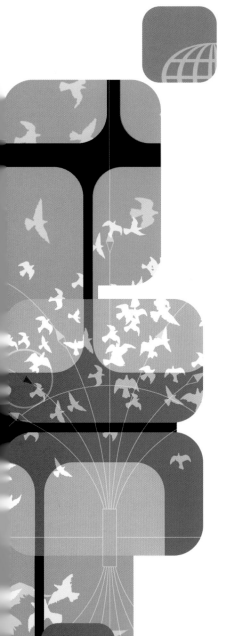

is constantly spewing out molten lava. This cools and sets in the magnetic field pattern of the seabed, giving the whales an important environmental cue. Interference from artificial magnetic fields puts whales at risk of being driven off course and beaching on some foreign shore.

The mystery of how birds navigate on long migratory flights has been solved by Wolfgang and Roswitha Wiltschko from the JW Goethe University, Frankfurt. They have discovered that bird navigation is a two stage process. First the birds determine the direction to their goal as a compass course, then they use an internal compass to convert it to a specific direction. The first description of an avian magnetic compass was for European robins (*Erithacus rubecula*), which migrate at night, probably making use of the dip angle as well as the field direction. Studies show that, for their first migratory journey, birds rely on innate information on the direction and distance of their route, and in later life they refine it with additional cues.

Homing pigeons are a different case from migrating birds. They find their way home over long distances across land and sea. How they do this is not fully understood, but it seems that their sensitivity to the Earth's magnetic field plays a part. In several similar episodes, homing pigeons in a race across Europe were exposed to an unusual magnetic solar storm. Thousands of them lost their way, and a good many were never seen again. From this evidence some have argued that their disorientation was due to the influence of the solar magnetic field affecting the magnetite in the pigeons' brains.

Migratory salmon return to the breeding river where they were born, even after several years at sea. Akira Yano of Chiba University, Japan followed the migratory response of chum salmon (*Oncorhynchus keta*) to the Earth's magnetic field. In an experiment in the waters off the Kuril islands he artificially modified this field using a radio-controlled electromagnet attached to the salmon's head. The data suggest that the fishes responded to the artificially induced magnetic field by altering their swimming depth.

Termite ants also exhibit sensitivity to magnetic fields. Gunther Becker, working in Berlin, showed that exposing termites to a magnetic field suppressed their gallery-building activity. The termites showed a preference for the geomagnetic field direction, and tried to build their galleries in the area furthest from the imposed artificial magnetic field.

endogenous fields

All living creatures depend on endogenous fields: internal electric and magnetic fields that send signals around the body to control nerves and muscles.

The human brain emits magnetic fields, measurable using MEG (Magnetoencephalogram) probes. The body's magnetic field was first measured in 1968 by David Cohen at the Massachusetts Institute of Technology, and the results were replicated in West Berlin in 1974. It has been suggested that the brain may control the body's chemistry through specific magnetic fields.

But the principal weak fields inside multi-cellular creatures are electric. The heartbeat rate is controlled by pulsating electric fields from the sino-atrial node of the heart. Electro-encephalogram (EEG) recordings measure the electric fields emitted by the brain, first discovered in human beings by Hans Berger in 1929 at the University of Jena, Germany. The pulses of different frequencies emitted by the brain are called alpha, beta, and theta rhythms. They must have a purpose, and seem to be individual for each person. The patterns also change when we are ill, and they increase dramatically during REM (rapid eye movement) sleep.

At Coghill Research Laboratories we found that each person's endogenous electric field provides a protective effect for the circulating white blood cells of his or her immune system (see page 39). The endogenous field of another human being had no protective effect: our endogenous fields are as individual to us as our DNA. So perhaps there is an information content in our brain rhythms so far unsuspected in biology.

Sensitivity to electric fields

At the Scripps Institute of Oceanography in La Jolla, California, a Dutch scientist Ad Kalmijn has been investigating how sharks can sense an electric field. When he brought the sharks to a spot on the shallow ocean bed with a chemical attractant

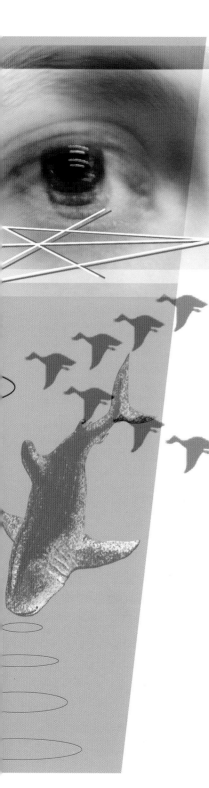

they naturally took bites at the area where the chemicals were, hoping for a food morsel. But Kalmijn had hidden several electric cables in the sand, and when he activated the cable a short distance away the shark immediately turned toward it and bit at it, even though it was concealed. When that circuit was switched off and another was activated, the shark immediately attacked the second cable. By gradually reducing the voltage Kalmijn was able to establish that sharks are sensitive to fields as low as a quarter millionth of a volt per metre – an exceptionally small field strength.

Kalmijn went on to identify a part of the brain, the ampullae of Lorenzini, as the shark's electric field sensors. Its use is obvious: the shark can sense its prey by the electric fields that all living creatures emit. Kalmijn still works on the sensitivities of fishes including large rays and has recently been asked to find ways of stopping sharks from biting at the submarine cables carrying electricity under the sea.

This sensitivity to electric fields is not confined to aquatic creatures. The land-based Australian duckbilled platypus can sense earthworms under the soil in the same manner, which enables it to find food.

Ulrich Warnke at the University of the Saarland has spent many years studying animal behavior patterns, particularly in ducks flying in convoy. He believes that each duck creates a high electric field through friction with the air, and that in the convoy the following bird positions itself to minimize electrical energy between itself and the bird in front. It is this positioning that creates the well known V-shaped flying formation.

In the same way, humans may also be able to detect others' electric fields (some call this field the aura). How many of us somehow know if a house we are visiting is empty before we knock on the door? Or know that someone is watching us from across the street, even without turning to look? Some scientists talk of psychic warfare, when malevolent people attempt to damage the endogenous field of their victim. This is quite in line with the laws of normal science: one electric field will disturb another.

This means in turn that our endogenous electric fields could be affected by external artificial electric fields, with adverse effects on the body's electrically controlled processes. These effects are discussed more in chapter two.

ions

Positive ions in the atmosphere have harmful effects on health, while negative ions are beneficial.

If an atom loses electrons (see page 20) it has more protons than electrons and so has an overall positive charge. Conversely, if an atom gains electrons, it has more electrons than protons and so is negatively charged. These charged particles are called ions, and all contain unpaired electrons.

Our bodies make extensive use of ions such as calcium (Ca^{++}), potassium (K^+), and sodium (Na^+) ions for transmitting electric signals between the brain and the nerves. So it is not surprising that large quantities of ions, whether natural or artificial in origin, can affect human health. One hypothesis is that such ions interfere with the body's own internal communications system.

Electric storms

Large numbers of ions are created naturally in an electric storm. How often have you heard people predict that a storm is coming "because I can feel it in my bones"? Their description is not merely a superstition. Water-laden clouds become negatively charged, due to friction between the water molecules and the air through which the cloud passes. Positive ions then accumulate beneath the cloud. As the clouds progress down the sky, these positive ions pile up and the wind begins to push them ahead of the clouds.

The Earth's surface is also negatively charged as a result of chemical reactions at its core. This high level of positive ions before a storm creates a distinct feeling of airlessness or stuffiness in the atmosphere. People with rheumatism or arthritis feel pain. Others call the air "close" or dead. Breathing does not seem to be so effective in these conditions, even though the amount of atmospheric oxygen is unchanged. Eventually the attraction between the negative and positive charges overcomes the air's resistance and the result is a flash

The moon's influence

The Earth is encompassed by the ionosphere, a mantle of ionized gas beneath which positive ions collect. At the full moon, the opposing gravitational forces of the sun and moon slightly squeeze the ionosphere. This pushes positive ions down toward the Earth, increasing the proportion of positive ions at the Earth's surface.

Conversely, at the new moon, the joint gravitational pull of sun and moon lifts the ionosphere slightly and reduces the concentration of positive ions beneath it.

or more of lightning. Thunder then rolls and down comes the rain. After the storm how clear and sweet the air appears! This is because the air is now surcharged with negative ions and the balance of negative and positive charges on the Earth's surface has been restored.

Effects of positive ions

At the full moon there are more positive ions at the Earth's surface (see opposite page) and people seem to suffer more stress. It has been well documented over hundreds of years that patients in mental hospitals become restless and excited at the time of the full moon; the word "lunatic" means one affected by the moon. There is also a significant increase in homicides, and generally disturbed social activity at such times.

A surfeit of positive ions also causes blood to flow more slowly (see left), and as a result oxygen in the blood is not carried to the muscles as efficiently, resulting in muscle pain.

Effects of negative ions

At the time of the new moon, when there are proportionally more negative ions at the Earth's surface, organic life flourishes and seeds grow better. In many cultures it is traditional to plant crops at this time.

Experiments in the work place with negative ionizers, electrically powered machines that generate and emit negative ions, show that an increased ratio of negative ions creates a calm atmosphere where work proceeds creatively. Office workers suffer less from headaches, fatigue, and absenteeism when a negative ionizer is running in the office, than when it is switched off unbeknown to the staff.

The role of magnets

The examples above show just some of the ways that unpaired electrons (in positive and negative ions) have effects on our bodies. Magnets "organize" such charged particles so that they all spin in the same direction (see page 20). All materials, including living organisms, are affected by magnets in this way. So you can begin to see how magnets have an effect on the body and can be used therapeutically. These uses are described more fully in chapter three.

Ion effects on blood flow

Red blood cells are slightly negatively charged, as are the surfaces of the blood vessels through which they flow, and for a very good reason. Because like charges repel each other, blood cells do not get attracted to the artery walls, or to each other, and so can flow smoothly along these narrow channels.

However, when we inhale positive ions these enter the lungs and then the bloodstream, where they lessen the negative charge on the blood cells. Thus the adhesion of blood cells to the vessel walls is increased and circulation efficiency decreases. In contrast, negative ions increase circulation efficiency.

geomagnetic variations

Anomalies in the Earth's magnetic and electric fields can have serious effects on health.

All life is bathed in natural low-frequency electromagnetic fields, generated principally by thunderstorm activity in the equatorial zones. These fields travel around the Earth between its surface and the ionosphere about 140 kilometres (88 miles) above, with a resonant frequency of around 7.8Hz. Called Schumann resonances, after WO Schumann who discovered them in 1954, these electromagnetic field resonances appear to be vital for human health. Astronauts deprived of this resonance as well as the geomagnetic field during space flights appear to suffer ill health, and to avoid this a simulation of these fields has been incorporated into space craft design.

Without the gentle vibration of the Schumann resonances our bodies do not heal as quickly: the resonances appear to stimulate cell growth and the healing of soft tissues. In an experiment in 1997, Dr Michael Heffernan of the Pain Control Clinic at Rockfort, Texas found that the electric frequency of soft tissue peaked during healing and returned to normal with resolution of the injury.

Geopathic stress

Given that our own bodies are using endogenous electric fields for a variety of reasons (see page 28), some still not charted, the arrival of stray electrons from an external electric field, whether natural or man-made, may well be an underlying cause of ill health. One natural cause of variations in the Earth's electric field is underground streams. Called black streams by dowsers, they have been identified as causes of ill health for hundreds of years. In the 1700s Lady Milbanke, a friend of the English poet Byron, discovered a young French boy whose sensitivity to underground flowing water was so acute that he cried out in pain when passing over such streams. Although

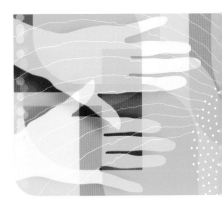

Case study

In 1999 Sergei Gerasimov, a Ukrainian doctor from Lviv State University, found a correlation between multiple sclerosis (MS) and the intensity of the local geomagnetic field. For example in Oslo, Norway, the high MS incidence of 60 per 10,000 coincides with a high geomagnetic field index at 154 units.

By contrast in Aden in the Yemen, the MS incidence is only 3 per 10,000 and the geo-field index is very low at only 12 units. Gerasimov suggests that since solar activity has a great impact on geomagnetic field perturbations, it could also indirectly affect MS epidemiological patterns.

such streams occur naturally, many more are created when water flows are conduited and led underground to allow for building on the land above.

The water in an underground stream is effectively flowing in an enclosed cylinder. Ragged electric fields are created as electrons are knocked off the water molecules through friction with the walls of the cylinders, and these fields can build up to extremely high levels.

More recently underground streams have been implicated in the incidence of chronic fatigue syndrome, as shown in the case studies, left. This modern disease, also called myalgic encephalitis (ME) or fibromyalgia, first appeared in the 1950s. We have to ask why these outbreaks did not occur before, since the conduits and underground streams had been there well before this date. The answer may lie in the first transmissions of radiated power for the domestic television from the nearby transmitters that were constructed around that time. It could well have been the combination of the electric fields from both these sources that had such devastating effects on health.

Case study

One of the first outbreaks of chronic fatigue syndrome occurred between July and October 1955 among nurses at the Royal Free Hospital, London. Some 255 nurses were admitted to hospital and others were also treated. Twelve patients developed the full syndrome, with symptoms including headache, depression and emotional instability, pains in the limbs, and dizziness. During the second and third weeks the patients became more severely ill, with facial paralysis, vertigo, and motor dysfunction.

The nurses' dormitory was on the Fleet Road, under which flows a powerful underground stream. The possibility that geopathic stress could be the underlying cause was not considered in the official investigation into the outbreak.

At the Middlesex Hospital, where another outbreak occurred in 1952, the nurses affected slept in a dormitory near a main storm-relief sewer. Similarly, in the 1970–71 outbreak at Great Ormond St Children's Hospital the nurses' dormitory was above an underground fresh-water conduit.

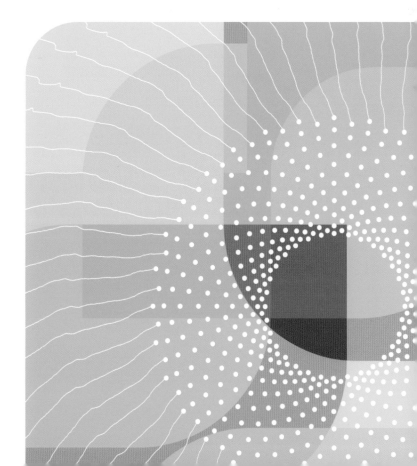

practical uses

Magnets' ability to speed liquid flow and prevent clogging has both health and technical benefits.

Saving fuel with magnets

The principle that magnets can align the spin state of unpaired electrons (see page 20) is used to improve fuel efficiency in combustion engines. The fuel is passed through a magnetic field of around 1400 gauss (140 millitesla) just before it enters the combustion chamber. The magnetic field distorts the tracks of the hydrogen ions and makes them spin in alignment, thus making them more available for reaction. The hydrocarbons in the fuel therefore flow more evenly and bond more readily with the carbon and oxygen in the air entering the carburation chamber, so combustion efficiency improves.

Several firms have pioneered this principle by offering magnets designed for attachment to fuel lines, claiming that this leads to a saving of more than 10 per cent in fuel costs, as well as a cleaner "burn". Despite controversy, a UK government study confirms magnet effectiveness. One private car hire firm in Shropshire fitted magnets to all its cars. The managing director reported a 10 per cent improvement in diesel fuel consumption, and gave an example of a Peugeot 309 GLi where the consumption of 15km per litre (42 miles per gallon) improved to 17km per litre (48mpg) when magnets were used.

Thus using magnets attached to the inflowing fuel line of a car is likely to reduce fuel costs, as well as harmful exhaust emissions.

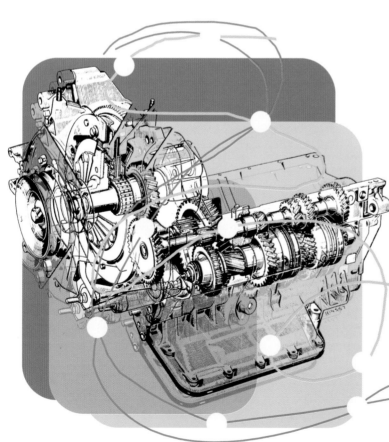

Using magnets in plumbing

Magnets can be used to prevent scale build-up and also to de-scale the interior of domestic and industrial water pipes. You will have seen how a kettle or coffee maker builds up a fur of calcium and other salts which eventually overwhelm the system. The same happens in water pipes. Applying magnets to the pipes creates a magnetic field that keeps the positively charged calcium ions in suspension, rather than allowing them to attach to the pipe walls.

Using magnets for pain relief

In the same way that they de-scale water pipes, magnets reduce clogging of the arteries and thus improve blood flow. How magnets have this effect is explained in more detail in chapter three (pages 74–5). Improved blood flow means that molecular oxygen and also the body's natural pain-relieving chemicals, the endorphins, can be transported through the bloodstream more efficiently.

A magnetic field affects the positively charged iron atoms in the blood's hemoglobin, enabling them to carry more oxygen to the muscles where it is needed. This improved bio-availability of oxygen means that the muscles can do more work before they become tired and start to ache.

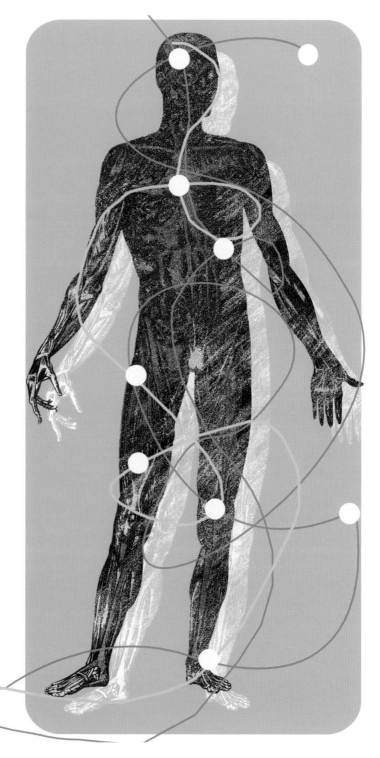

chapter 2
your magnetic health

In the past fifty years, developments in electrically powered technology have revolutionized our lives. As a result our environment is bathed in man-made alternating electric and magnetic fields.

This chapter explores the possible negative effects of these artificial fields on health and wellbeing and offers practical advice on minimizing exposure to them.

Domestic electric and magnetic fields vary greatly and can be affected by factors such as the layout of electric circuits, how electrical appliances are wired, and where they are sited. Simple practical steps show how to reduce your exposure to alternating fields while you sleep, when your body may be most affected by these potentially damaging fields. Room-by-room guides outline further steps to protect yourself in every area of your home.

The chapter ends with a look at sources of high electric fields in the wider environment, such as high voltage power lines, electric train lines, and cellphone transmitters. There are recommendations for safe distances for housing from such installations, and of other measures you can take to protect yourself from their effects.

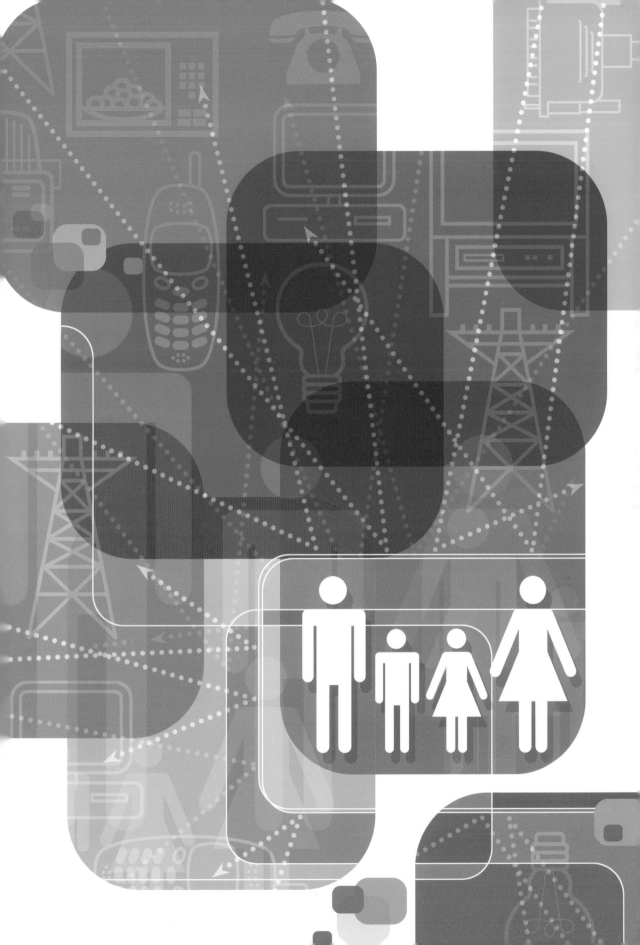

our electric environment

We are surrounded by electric fields, both natural and artificial.

Electric storms create a natural electric field, when the attraction between the positively charged clouds and the negatively charged Earth's surface eventually leads to a flash of lightning (see page 31). These electrical changes have noticeable effects on health.

Other naturally occurring electric fields are beneficial to health. Sea air is bracing and invigorating because it is negatively charged. As the waves crash on the shore, electrons are dislodged from their atoms and form clouds of negative ions. Mountain air has also long been considered to have health-giving qualities. This is because of the negative ions that accumulate around mountain peaks.

But most of the electric fields that envelop us are not naturally occurring. We are surrounded by a cocktail of different electromagnetic waves – radio waves transmitting television and radio, microwaves from satellites, electric fields from overhead cables. These all contribute to a background level of electrical activity, measurable even in unspoiled and uninhabited areas of the countryside. Since we are not all dying like flies, it seems that low-level electric fields are not too harmful to us. But within our homes, near high-voltage power lines, electrified railway lines, or cellphone transmitter masts, the electric fields can be much higher.

At what level do these electric fields become harmful? Research is beginning to provide some answers to this question, though these are not yet incorporated into official thinking. The exposure guidelines of the US National Council for Radiation Protection suggest that a safe level is 5,000 volts per metre for the general public. This is the same as the European guidelines. However, the UK National Radiological Protection Board (NRPB) suggest that fields can reach a level of 12,000 volts per metre before any investigation is needed

Case study

In the early 1950s the US Embassy in Moscow was found to have the highest level of cancer incidence per head of population in the world. This prompted the investigation known as Project Pandora, which found that the immune systems of the Embassy staff had been seriously compromised, possibly by weak microwave radiations designed to collect bugging information. The exposure to Embassy staff was at a level of around $18\mu W/cm^2$ (microwatts per square centimetre).

Subsequent studies have confirmed that one important adverse effect of microwave radiation is that it damages immune system cells.

into health effects. In Russia the safe level is judged to be just 500 volts per metre. This variation illustrates how uncertain the experts are about the exposure standards.

Effects of electric fields on the body

Mankind has evolved in the presence of the Earth's static magnetic field, so the body's endogenous electric fields have developed to work perfectly within it. But alternating magnetic and electric fields, generated by modern electrical appliances, are relatively new, and their effects can be harmful.

Unorganized electrons within the body, known as free radicals, can damage cells by interfering with energy synthesis at a cellular level. Enzymes and hormones such as melatonin play a vital role in mopping up these dangerous unpaired electrons. But a strong electric field and its accompanying alternating magnetic field can distort electron flows in the body so much that these inbuilt safety mechanisms are overloaded and unable to cope.

In an alternating electric field, electrons are pulsed in waves. The direction of the current changes 50 times per second in the UK, or 60 times per second in the US (see page 25). The rhythm of these waves can interfere with the rhythms of the body's endogenous field, such as the heartbeat. Also, research shows that the endogenous electric fields are important for the cellular immune system, and disturbing this natural mechanism adversely affects the immune system's competence.

Effects of magnetic fields

The alternating current that powers our domestic electrical appliances generates an extremely low frequency (ELF) field. In these fields there is no simple relationship between the magnetic and electric components, which need to be measured separately. Most research on the effects of overhead power lines has focused only on the magnetic fields, so the hazards of the electric field have not shown up.

The alternating magnetic field component of an alternating electric field penetrates the body tissue and is capable of inducing an electric field within it (see page 24). This may not necessarily be harmful – in chapter three we explore how such induced fields can heal, using precise frequencies that either mimic or interrupt the brain's electrical pulses. But in general, it is better to protect yourself from outside electric disturbances.

Research

In a study in 1998 at Coghill Research Laboratories we took a culture of lymphocytes from one person and divided it into four separate containers. Lymphocytes are cells which travel through the blood and attack foreign agents. One batch was connected to the endogenous electric field of the lymphocyte donor via a gold wire between the person's skin and the container. One batch was connected to the endogenous field of another person, one to an artificial electric field, and one left as a control.

The experiment was repeated several times, with consistent results. The cells exposed to the donor's electric field remained viable significantly longer than those in the other batches. Indeed, the artificial electric field, and the other person's endogenous field, had adverse effects on the cells. In other words, the donor's endogenous signals were somehow important for the wellbeing of the cells.

We concluded that a donor's endogenous electric fields have a biological purpose and are important for the cellular immune system.

domestic electric fields

Electric field levels in the home can vary greatly, depending on the electrical appliances used and how they are positioned.

Our homes are full of electrical appliances: from work saving devices such as refrigerators and washing machines, to appliances for entertainment and work such as videos, CD players, computers, cellphones, and fax machines. We light our rooms, cook our food, and heat our domestic hot water and our rooms with electricity.

All these appliances generate electric fields. So do the electric wiring circuits in the house, the electricity supply cables that enter the house, and others that pass close by. Outside, high voltage power lines passing overhead on pylons, radio and television signals, and the signals from cellphone masts all contribute to the electric field in the home.

In most homes the background level of the electric field is between 1 and 10 volts per metre (Vm^{-1}), which seems to be safe. Studies suggest that adverse effects seem to occur in fields of above $20Vm^{-1}$, compared with the NRPB recommendations of $12,000Vm^{-1}$ (see page 38). Such high fields are not often found in homes, but can occur close to electrical appliances. Also, each appliance generates its own field and these may interact in quite complex ways. The field in one position may change quite abruptly if some distant appliance is switched on. I once found that the electric fields in a bedroom suddenly changed around seven o'clock each night when they became very high, then collapsed again each morning just after dawn. Try as I might, I could not locate the origin of these changes. Finally it transpired they were being caused by the automatic switching on and off of the street lighting in the road outside at dusk and dawn.

Another bizarre example of the quixotic nature of electric fields was when I left an experiment running with a measuring meter on my living room table, and went to bed. The meter had a built-in audible alarm which sounded if the electric field exceeded certain levels. In the night I switched on my bedside lamp and suddenly heard the meter's alarm ringing on the floor below. When I switched off the lamp it stopped. A few more switches determined that by switching on my bedside lamp I was somehow increasing the electric field in the living room on the floor below.

Because of these interactions, the only way to know if you are being exposed to unusual electric fields in any part of your home is to monitor the location continually over a period of time. Spot measurements will not give an accurate picture. Many of the meters available only measure the magnetic component, so make sure that you use a meter that measures both the electric and magnetic fields (see resources on page 120).

The effect of metals
Metals conduct electricity, so if a metal object is placed in an electric field, the field will be conducted to each part of it. On several occasions I have found cases of chronic fatigue syndrome (ME) or childhood leukemia where the patient slept on a brass bed, positioned near an electric field source. As a result the bed produced a high electric field. The effect can be similar for mattresses with inbuilt metal springs. Metal radiators also conduct an electric field, so avoid putting beds near these.

This problem of conductive materials can complicate the profile of domestic electric fields enormously. In some homes partition walls are made from drywall or plasterboard insulated with aluminium foil. The electric wiring runs along the foil, which conducts its electric field through the foil, along the whole length of the wall.

Seasonal variations
Several years ago the UK National Grid published a seasonal profile of domestic electrical use for different types of home. This showed that there was a significant fall off in electricity consumption during the summer months (though they omitted August, when the measuring team went on vacation!) and a peak in February. Similar studies in Australia have shown that the pattern is reversed there to correspond with the seasons in the southern hemisphere. In some parts of the US, electricity usage actually increases during the summer months through use of air conditioners.

Case study
I once visited the home of a famous author who was suffering from chronic fatigue syndrome (CFS). She had written several best selling novels on an old computer whose screen emitted high electric fields and I suspected this was the root cause of her illness. Though I persuaded her to replace the computer for a low radiation model, I could not get her to abandon her electric blanket in favour of a down comforter or duvet. I was not surprised that although her CFS symptoms abated after the change of computer, she still suffers from the condition.

Research
Our laboratory measured the electric fields in the bedrooms of 60 people with chronic fatigue syndrome, and found that they all had a clearly elevated exposure to electric fields, compared with matched controls. Many lived in houses on the corner of a street and were therefore exposed to underground cables running along two sides of their homes.

domestic magnetic fields

The electric wiring circuits could be the cause of high magnetic fields in your home.

In most homes the level of the alternating magnetic field is around 40–50 nanotesla (nT). The sources of these magnetic fields are the same as for electric fields such as electrical appliances, or power lines outside, since all electric fields have a magnetic component. In studies of measured magnetic fields the adverse effects start to appear when the levels are around five times the norm, at around 200nT, but they are still weak associations and don't really strengthen until above 400nT. Not many homes have such levels, except quite close to some domestic appliances, and only then when these appliances are switched on. The table on the opposite page gives some examples of magnetic fields generated by typical domestic electrical equipment.

Another common cause of high magnetic fields in the home is unbalanced currents. Around any current-carrying wire there is a magnetic field (see page 24). When the outward (live) wire of any circuit is close to the wire returning from the appliance to the mains fuse box to complete the circuit, the magnetic fields from the wires tend to cancel each other out. To ensure this, many distribution cables are twisted together to form aerially bundled cable (known as ABC cabling). However, if the outward and returning wires are far apart, this creates an unbalanced circuit, and the magnetic fields can be high. A typical example is a circuit up a staircase, where the stair light can be switched on from either the bottom or the top of the stairs.

Normally the electricity supply circuit to homes ensures that the outward live and returning neutral are kept close together and follow one route from the transformer supplying the electricity to the homes they serve. Unbalanced ground return currents can occur if the route from the transformer turns a sharp angle, as well as in porous ground, where the home's electrical earthing system lets the neutral carry the returning current through the ground back to the transformer, rather than through the neutral cable. In this way a large ground loop can be formed, and in this the magnetic fields are often very high.

Electricians test to make sure this isn't happening by measuring the current to see if it is unbalanced. If a ground current is present it must be located and eliminated.

I was once asked to check the computer screens in a training school where the trainees found that half a dozen of their computers always seemed to leave them with a headache. This was strange because all the machines were identical models, but these six had been added a few months after the first batch. When I investigated I found that the additional cable had been incorrectly wired, so the live and neutral were reversed. This meant that the six new machines were giving off much higher magnetic fields than their earlier identical companions.

Even wiring an electric plug the wrong way round can create an unbalanced circuit to an appliance, perhaps resulting in unusually high magnetic fields. Always follow the manufacturer's instructions for wiring plugs and throughout the circuit, and have electrical fittings installed by a qualified electrician to ensure that you avoid such problems.

Field strengths
This table shows the magnetic and electric field strengths of common appliances at typical user distances.

	Magnetic field strength	Electric field strength	User distance
Television	70nT	$20Vm^{-1}$	100cm (39in)
Electric coffee maker/kettle	50nT	$6Vm^{-1}$	50cm (19.5in)
Vacuum cleaner	780nT	$8Vm^{-1}$	50cm (19.5in)
Hairdryer	17,440nT	$95Vm^{-1}$	5cm (2in)
	120nT	$11Vm^{-1}$	50cm (19.5in)
Washing machine	960nT	$15Vm^{-1}$	50cm (19.5in)
Iron	1840nT	$9Vm^{-1}$	5cm (2in)
Clock radio	50nT	$20Vm^{-1}$	50cm (19.5in)
Microwave oven	1660nT	$3Vm^{-1}$	50cm (19.5in)
Central heating pump	210nT	$15Vm^{-1}$	50cm (19.5in)

protecting yourself

Simple steps can minimize your exposure to harmful electric fields, and reduce the risks to your health.

We all enjoy the benefits of modern electrical appliances, and most of us would not wish to manage without them for longer than a couple of days. Yet evidence suggests that you could suffer ill health after prolonged exposure to the electric fields these appliances emit. Following the four practical steps outlined below will protect you from some of the harmful effects of electric fields in your home.

1. Avoid putting beds near electrical appliances
Where you sleep is important. Most adults sleep for around eight hours in every twenty four, and children for even longer. So if you are sleeping in an electric field you will be exposing yourself to its potentially harmful effects for long periods. Some scientists believe that the body's cellular repair takes place while we sleep. Alternating electric and magnetic fields can interfere with these delicate processes (see page 28). For the same reason, armchairs and sofas should also be placed away from electrical appliances.

One electrical instrument that you may not consider to be an appliance is the electricity meter, which measures the amount of electricity you use in your home. These constantly use current and can generate high fields, even on the other side of the wall to which they are attached. So check the position of this meter before you position your furniture.

2. Avoid sleeping near electric heaters
In the UK and some other countries, electricity tariffs are considerably cheaper at night than during the day. To take advantage of this some electric heaters are designed to run overnight. Electric storage heaters heat up the stones inside them overnight and release this heat during the day. Similarly,

Case study

A national US newspaper asked me to research why a cluster of 19 infants had died in a small area of California, below a newly erected radio and microwave transmitter site. In almost all the cases the electric field in the sleeping area was very high, except one, where it was perfectly normal.

I decided to investigate that case further. The mother explained that she had a full term normal birth, and the baby was healthy. When the baby was six weeks old they went for a vacation in a log cabin at Lake Tahoe in Northern California. The weather turned cold, so at night they placed the baby's crib near the electric fire.

After a week they noticed she was snuffling and was developing a cold, so they turned up the electric fire. After 10 days she was clearly very unwell, and so they abandoned the vacation and returned home, where she died the night they got back.

electric heaters in hot water tanks heat the water during the night. Anything placed near them is exposed to their adverse effects, so the obvious solution is not to place your bed near either. Think twice about putting a baby's crib in the bedroom housing the hot water tank and electric water heater, even though this room may be comfortable and warm.

If you need to use an electric heater overnight, place it as far as possible from the bed, so it is heating the air of the room and not you directly.

3. Switch off and unplug appliances after use

Whenever current flows through an appliance there is an electric field around it. In some appliances the on/off switch is located in the wiring circuit after live current has passed through the appliance, so even when it is switched off current flows through it and generates an electric field.

The problem can be solved by always pulling out the plug from the electric socket after switching off the appliance.

4. Keep your distance from electrical appliances

The table on page 43 gives field values for a number of household appliances, based on a typical user distance. As you move farther away from the source, the strength of the field decreases (see page 23), so it makes sense not to sit too close to the television, for example.

Handheld tools such as electric drills, sanders, hedge trimmers, or hairdryers, generate high electric fields and are held close to the body. Often we only use them for a minute or two anyway, but for bigger jobs, such as sanding a floor, you may be exposed for much longer. You may also use such machines in your work. If you need to use hand tools for more than an hour at a time, have a rest for at least ten minutes every hour.

Follow the simple steps outlined, but keep a sense of proportion. The stress of worrying excessively about electromagnetic fields could in the long term have more serious health effects than the fields themselves.

Pages 46–53 give a room-by-room breakdown of the most common electrical appliances used in the home, with specific tips on how to use them safely and limit exposure to their electric fields.

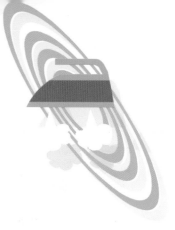

the kitchen

Protect yourself from electric fields generated by kitchen appliances.

Modern kitchens contain a large number of electric machines and gadgets and also tend to be the "hub" of the home where people eat and congregate, as well as cook.

Iron
In common with any other hand-held electrical appliance, this generates a high electric field and is held close to the body. Try to limit your exposure: if ironing for long periods be sure to take a 10-minute break every hour.

Electric sockets
There is inevitably an electric field around these. You are unlikely to spend much time near them in the kitchen, but in other rooms make sure you keep your armchair or bed away from them.

Radio
The electric fields generated by radios are not very high, so there are unlikely to be any adverse effects.

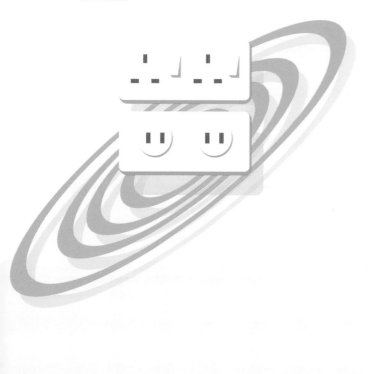

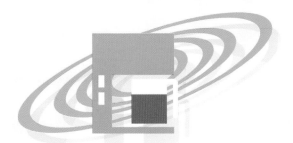

Electric coffee maker

There is no evidence that boiling water by electricity affects the water in any way that is harmful to health. Coffee makers that keep the coffee warm give off high fields, so don't place them where you are likely to sit for long periods. Incidentally, caffeine (like nicotine and alcohol) penetrates the blood–brain barrier, affecting immune competence. Electromagnetic fields and radiation may exacerbate the effect.

Refrigerator and freezer

These appliances need to run all the time to maintain a steady temperature, so although their fields are not high, they are constant. Ensure that they are not situated on the opposite side of the wall to your bed or armchair.

Electric hotplate and oven

These give off very high fields when heating food. You may have to stand close to the hotplate while stirring a sauce, for example, but in general keep away from them while they are switched on.

Microwave oven

All microwave ovens are tested to make sure that the external exposure levels are less than 5000mW/cm^2. However serious adverse health effects have been reported from exposure at only 18μW/cm^2 (see page 38). Do not stand in front of the oven while it is cooking, as the electric fields are enormous next to the appliance, often at eye (and therefore brain) level.

Unlike an electric field, microwave radiation does not stop when the source is turned off. So follow the instructions and leave microwaved food for 5 minutes after cooking before eating it.

the living room

Protect yourself from electric fields where you relax.

Subdued lighting, a warm fire, soft music, and the calming influence of swimming fish all create a relaxing atmosphere. But the appliances that generate this ambience also generate electric fields.

CD and cassette player
Some people prefer to leave these switched on all the time, to avoid power surges that could damage the circuits. If you do this, make sure your player is not placed next to your sofa where you spend time relaxing.

Table lamp
A lamp with a metal base creates very high fields. There is anecdotal evidence of people suffering frequent migraines or headaches after sitting reading for long periods by such lamps. When the lamps were replaced with wooden ones, the headaches ceased.

Extension cord or cable
Always unwind an extension cord fully before use, or the fields from the coil will be very high, and may even be a fire risk.

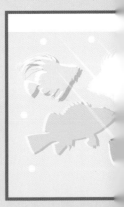

Standard lamp

As for table lamps: avoid placing lamps made of metal, especially brass, near your armchair or anywhere you rest for long periods.

Fish tank

The pump or heater is usually powered by a transformer and the electric field from this is transmitted through the water in the tank, so the entire fish tank can become a source of enormous electric fields in the living room. Locate your tank away from places where you may sit for long periods.

Adjustable light switch

This type of light switch gives out very high electric fields unless it has a well earthed brass coverplate. Ensure that your sofa or armchair (or in the bedroom, your bed) is not placed near the switch.

Radiant electric fire

The fields around these can be high, so do not sit directly in front of them. It makes sense to heat the room air, not yourself directly. (See case study on page 45.)

Television

The electric field is high right next to the screen, maybe as much as 50 volts per metre. However at 2.5m (8ft) away from the screen it will have fallen to around background levels. So don't sit too close to the screen – children in particular tend to – and use the remote control to change channels.

the bedroom

Protect yourself from electric fields where you sleep.

We probably spend more time in our bedrooms than in any other room. Electric fields in the bedroom affect you as you sleep, but there are simple ways to reduce your exposure to them.

Negative ionizer

This is the one electrical appliance that is beneficial in the bedroom, as long as it is placed away from the bed on the other side of the room. The negative ions improve circulation and the availability of energy-giving oxygen in the blood (see page 31).

Electric blanket

These emit some of the highest fields of all, very close to the body. If you leave the blanket on all night you are exposed to those fields for many hours at a time. In some electric blankets the wiring circuit is arranged so that the switch is located after the live current has passed through the blanket. In this case simply switching off at the switch on the supply cord, or relying on the time switch, may not be sufficient to avoid exposure to the electric field. The safest way is to use the blanket to warm the bed and then pull the plug out of the socket at the wall before you get in.

Hairdryer

Along with heated hair brushes and hot rollers, these have high electric fields and are held very close to the head. Limit your exposure as far as possible.

Electrically powered shower

The electric field of this shower unit is high only while the shower is running. Therefore it is unlikely to have harmful effects on your health.

Baby monitor

These are of two types: electric powered or wireless units. Both transmit at radio frequencies, and the electric powered type also generate electric fields. They are often left on all night so that parents can be sure to hear their baby cry from another room. Place the monitor at the other side of the room, as far from the baby as possible, where it should still pick up sounds adequately.

Clock radio and alarm

These are often placed right next to the pillow, and because of their function are always switched on. They are a common source of chronic exposure at close range to alternating currents and electric fields. Place the clock on the other side of the room so that you are not sleeping in its electric field. Then you will need to get out of bed to stop the alarm each morning, ensuring that it really wakes you up.

Bedside lamp

Lamps with metal bases give off very high electric fields, so choose one with a ceramic or wooden base.

the workroom and study

Protect yourself from electric fields in your work environment.

The majority of homes now own a personal computer and other electrical appliances traditionally thought of as office equipment, such as answer phones and fax machines. And with more people working from home, this trend is set to continue. The workroom may also be a place where children do their homework, surf the internet, or play computer games.

Cordless phone
These use much lower frequencies than cellphones, and no studies to date have reported any elevated ill health incidence from their use. However the newer digital (DECT) phones radiate all the time, and they may be a cause of headaches. It is probably best to restrict their use as far as possible.

Cellphone or mobile telephone
These transmit and receive low power microwaves, which can be absorbed by the body's tissues. No study has shown any adverse effects from short duration calls, so if you use a cellphone for less than five minutes per call you are unlikely to suffer harm. Headaches after using a cellphone are the first sign from the brain that all is not well.

Computer screen
Workstations are usually only 50cm (19.5in) from the operator's face, hands, and upper limbs so electric field exposure is high. The recommended exposure limits for screens are much lower than for electric field exposure generally, but also vary according to different authorities. In New York the safe level for computers for use in public is 250nT or 25 volts per metre at 30cm (12in) from the screen. Elsewhere in the US the same levels apply at 50cm (19.5in) distance. In the UK and Europe the new TCO-95 guidelines are even lower, and most screens these days are designed for low radiation.

Radiation screens, available from most office equipment suppliers, give extra protection provided they are earthed so that any stray electrons are conducted away. Some claim that a certain cactus (*Peruvianus*) placed near computer terminals helps ward off their rays, and others swear by large quartz crystals. These won't harm you, and may look attractive as well.

Laptop computer

Laptop screens do not emit radiation, but if you are running a laptop computer on electric power the last place to use it is on your lap. Instead use the computer on a table to increase your distance and shielding from its electric fields.

Most laptops have a separate transformer attached by a 1m (3ft) cable, so place this as far as possible from your body to use the appliance without serious exposure to electric current.

Computer games

These games are linked to a computer monitor or television, and children can play them for hours at a time, sitting close to the screen. It is the screen that is the hazard, rather than the computer element (see television, page 49). The answer is to use a long lead so that players sit at least 2.5m (3 yards) from the screen, and limit their use.

Answering machines

These are usually powered by a transformer attached to the plug. It is this transformer that is responsible for their high fields, not the instrument itself. If the power point is down near the floor, not too close to areas where you sit for any length of time, the fields should not cause problems.

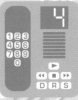

Desk lamp

The enormous fields that some metal lamps can emit are astonishing, especially the halogen type. This is because the electric cord or cable does not have an earth wire, so watch out for any other appliances wired similarly. Avoid using one on your office or home desk.

Fax machine

As with the answering machine, the transformer is the main source of electric fields. Avoid putting your most comfortable chair right next to the fax machine power point. If you do not spend time near it, the fields should not cause problems.

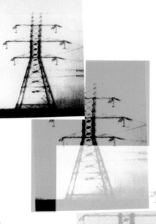

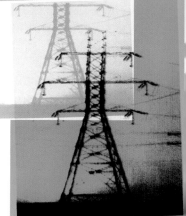

power lines

Ever since high voltage lines first appeared in the 1950s, concerns have been raised about their possible adverse effects on health.

Of the dozen or so epidemiological studies of childhood leukemia in relation to power lines, only two concluded there was no association between the two, and these were both funded by the power utility companies (Rhode Island 1980; Yorkshire 1985). Moreover in both these cases the authors eventually had to admit that their study design was flawed, and could not be used to conclude that no association existed.

The difference between electric and magnetic fields has been exploited by the power utility companies in their attempts to deny any biological effects from power lines. Their studies have mainly only measured the magnetic fields and not the electric component. When Coghill Research Laboratories measured the electric field in leukemic children's homes a very strong association emerged. This research was published in 1996, and the same effect showed up in a Canadian occupational study later the same year. More recently research has linked other kinds of symptoms with high voltage (HV) power lines, such as depressive illness and suicide, headache, epilepsy, dizziness, and heart conditions.

Before you can assess the effects of a given power line, you need to know the voltage it carries. In the UK the common voltages are 275,000 and 400,000 volts; in the US they are slightly different: 220,000 and 375,000 volts. In Russia some lines have voltages as high as 750,000 volts. Until recently in the UK, except for Scotland, the voltage carried was posted on each pylon, but this practice has been discontinued.

The strength of the magnetic fields from a power line depends on how much current is flowing. Using a field meter I was able to show one worried group of residents with a power line passing through their housing estate that the line was not actually being energized, and so there was no

Case study

In December 1999 the results of a national study of several thousand children with leukemia in the UK announced that there was no excess risk for children sleeping in higher than normal magnetic fields. But the promoters of the study did not tell the public what they had discovered regarding the safety of electric fields. These results would be published later.

The same week a study by Professor Denis Henshaw and colleagues at Bristol University reported that the risk of cancer from power line electric fields could be twice the average. They suggest that the free electrons in these electric fields are breathed into the lungs and act as damaging free radicals (see page 39).

Case study

In the village of Dalmally, 64 km (40 miles) from Glasgow, the 36-home community is divided by a 275kV line taking and returning current to the UK's largest hydro electric power scheme at nearby Cruachan. In this community eight people died of cancer in five years, all living in two streets by the line. There were also three non-fatal breast cancers and three deaths from motor neurone disease in this period. The incidence of these disorders in such a small community is well above national averages.

Case study

Ferndown, Dorset, is about 20 km (12 miles) from Bournemouth on the south coast of England. The town is traversed by a number of power lines supplying Bournemouth's electricity. In Ferndown there has been an elevated incidence of childhood leukemia for some years: a cluster of 60 cases in a population of 200,000 compared with the average of 400 cases annually in the whole of the country.

magnetic field to worry about. Although it is the electric field component that is most harmful, alternating magnetic fields can induce electrical currents in the body that interfere with the endogenous fields, with adverse effects.

When a power line is energized there will be an electric field even if there is no current consumption. The same thing applies to the wiring in your home: plug in your electric iron and you have created an electric field around the cable even without switching it on.

Several power lines together

Often HV lines are in groups and their combined magnetic fields increase with the extra load. Sometimes two or more lines join together, creating higher electric and magnetic fields between them through the addition of the two fields. We have noticed that the incidence of ill health is much higher in areas between two power lines that join at an angle of less than 90 degrees. This is illustrated by the case studies, left.

Electricity transformers and substations

High voltage cables carry power to substations, where the voltage is converted to a lower level, suitable for domestic use, by a transformer. The transformers are usually metal clad, so all the electric field is contained within the casing and the external electric field is normally minimal. These transformers are often situated close to houses. In the UK the NRPB guidelines suggest that, for safety, they should be at least 25 metres (27 yards) from houses (see page 59).

In the US, and more rarely in the UK, small distribution line transformers are often mounted on poles near houses and are therefore much nearer bedrooms and sleeping areas. An epidemiological study by Nancy Wertheimer and Ed Leeper in Denver, Colorado in 1979, found a dramatic increase in the risk of childhood leukemia near these transformers and the high level of electric cabling associated with them.

electrified train lines

Overhead lines on electrified railways have been linked to health problems.

In the mid 1980s a group of scientists in San Francisco were monitoring local changes in electric fields in an effort to link these to earthquake activity. They hammered two nails into a large tree in the hills above the city, one a metre (three feet) or so above the other, and their delicate instruments continuously sampled the field between the nails. They soon noticed a curious regular disturbance, which they could not link to any obvious source. Because the disturbance was clearly less obvious at weekends and also slowed considerably overnight, they guessed it must be man-made.

Then, by chance, one scientist saw the instrument react exactly at the moment when the Bay Area Rapid Transport (BART) train stopped at a station far below and 14 kilometres (9 miles) distant. The electric surge from the trains was the culprit! As the ensuing *New Scientist* article put it: if trains can do that to trees, what can they be doing to us?

Sudden infant death syndrome

In London three mainline stations, Euston, St Pancras, and King's Cross are adjacent to each other. Every day hundreds of trains arrive and depart from these two stations, along electrified lines through the borough of Camden. In the mid 1980s I carried out a survey of sudden infant death syndrome (SIDS, or cot death) in Camden and also three other central London boroughs (Islington, Hackney, and Tower Hamlets). I was appalled to see that SIDS occurred much more frequently near sources of electric field disturbance such as the overground electrified railway lines, underground train lines, high voltage power lines, and similar installations. The nearer the infants had lived to them, the younger they had died. The evidence was statistically overwhelming, and

Case study

No one has ever plotted cancers or SIDS cases in London in relation to train lines, but Dr Egon Eckert did so for several cities, including Philadelphia and Hamburg. These results were published in a German medical journal in 1976. He claimed to show a significant correlation of SIDS with proximity to railway or tramway lines, especially where they crossed at acute angles. However the authorities have completely ignored his work, as well as his requests for further investigation, because the socio-economic implications are enormous.

questions about it were asked in the UK Parliament in 1989, but despite promises, nothing was ever done.

The following year, the infant son of a well known TV presenter, Anne Diamond, died from SIDS. In order to be near the Camden TV studio for her early morning presentations, Ms Diamond had moved to a house less than 100 metres (110 yards) from the electrified railway at Camden. I already knew of a half dozen similar SIDS cases in the surrounding streets, from the north London coroner's records I had consulted during the study.

Subsequently Anne Diamond was instrumental in a nationwide campaign to give better advice to parents, and SIDS death figures for the UK have since declined, though even today some ten infants in the UK and more in the US die each week. I believe that some of those deaths originate from exposure to high voltage power lines, such as train lines, since a human infant's brain is not able to withstand their onslaught.

Isolating causes of ill health

Also in London, in 1986, a housing association asked me to investigate the likely impact of a new electrified line linking the Paddington railway terminus to Heathrow Airport, which would pass directly behind their apartment block.

In this block one little boy had already contracted leukemia. When I visited I noticed that all the power boxes for the apartments were in the basement walls, grouped in just a few areas. With the help of neighbours' memories I constructed a map of the cancers in the block over the years, and was able to show that these were most prevalent near the mains supply boxes, gradually lessening in incidence with distance, and with fewest cases on the top floor.

Part of my advice was that these boxes be dispersed more widely, and not placed on walls in sleeping areas. But I could think of nothing to protect the residents from the electric surges from a train line, except to move home.

This story illustrates how it can be misleading to focus exclusively on one possible cause of electropollution, rather than looking at the bigger picture.

cellphone transmitters

With astonishing speed a new and important source of electromagnetic radiation has spread around the globe.

In 1993 the World Health Organization (WHO) did not even consider cellphone use in their publication on electromagnetic field health issues. By January 2000 the UK had over twenty four million cellphone users, with seventy five million in the US, and at least 500 million worldwide.

Acoustic neuroblastoma cancers are increasingly being associated with cellphone use. Research to date has not shown adverse effects from short calls (see page 52), but if you have to make longer calls, you could try fitting a shield or device to the phone to reduce the amount of radiation reaching your head (see resources on page 120). Attaching an earpiece allows you to make calls hands free with the phone farther away from your body, but these accessories have not yet been properly evaluated for health risks. They may provide a good pathway for adverse fields and radiations to arrive at your ear.

If you choose to walk round with the most radiative domestic device ever invented held to your ear, that is your choice. But I have had countless complaints from communities plagued by the sudden appearance of the cellphone transmitter masts, or "base stations" as they are called, which expose everyone in the area to radio frequency and extra low frequency (ELF) signals. But despite evidence that such installations cause ill health in the local population, even the latest WHO research initiative does not regard base station health effects as a priority.

Base station signals

A geographical area is divided into zones called "cells". These can be as small as one kilometre (half a mile) across in busy areas, up to a maximum of around 80 kilometres (50 miles).

Research

In Lund, Sweden, Per Salford and colleagues showed that cellphone frequency microwaves affected the blood–brain barriers of animals exposed to them. The blood–brain barrier protects the brain from infection.

At the University of Washington, Seattle, Henry Lai and NP Singh demonstrated that microwaves could break single and double strands of DNA faster than repair enzymes could restore the vital links and avoid mutation.

There is a base station in the middle of each of these cells. Suppose you use your cellphone to call your sister on her cellphone. Your phone makes contact with the nearest base station, which transmits your call via the terrestrial phone network to the base station nearest to your sister's cellphone. This then transmits the call to your sister's cellphone.

So when a cellphone is switched on, it constantly sends an ELF signal to the base station of its current cell area, to signal its whereabouts. The base station returns similar signals, which have a typical pulse of 217Hz in the UK, or 50Hz in the US. Both these frequencies are close to the delicate frequencies used by the brain to signal to the body's cells, the body's endogenous fields (see page 28). It is a reasonable hypothesis that artificial radiations could interfere with brain–cell communications, just as early radio stations caused interference before radio frequency bands were regulated.

Research

Helen Dolk of the London School of Tropical Medicine produced evidence, albeit weak, of a higher incidence of adult leukemias near TV transmitters, and in Sydney a smaller study found the same. In a three-university Chinese study of over 1000 children and army cadets, those living nearest radio and microwave sources were found to have impaired immune systems.

A Latvian study also found that children who had spent several years living in the beam of a powerful radio-location system had significantly poorer memories and reaction times compared with pupils living nearby but not exposed.

In Bern, Switzerland, a shortwave transmitter was closed down after a study showed that ill health (headaches, general tiredness) increased with proximity to the mast.

The effects of base stations

The few studies that have looked into the possible adverse health effects of cellphone masts and base stations (see left) show that we are right to be concerned. These studies are not enough for conclusive proof, but they have been sufficient to stop the approval of base station installations in a number of cases worldwide. In some other cases transmitter masts have been relocated after this evidence was provided to local authorities. The internet boasts sites for action groups in many countries who can share their knowledge with communities faced with planning applications for cellphone masts.

Taking the evidence of these studies together gives a power density threshold for reported ill health. By converting this into typical safe distances (using NRPB figures) and then dividing by ten to give a clear safety margin, I have devised my own rule of thumb that no mast should be placed within 200 metres (220 yards) of any inhabited building, and certainly not – until we know more about the effects – on school buildings. If a new pharmaceutical were placed straight onto the market without full testing for toxicity there would be a public and media outcry, yet this is precisely what the telecommunication industry has done with base stations. Areas exposed chronically to a nearby cellphone base station have usually had little say in the decision, which is patently unfair.

protection from HV lines

How can we protect ourselves from the electric fields around high voltage power lines?

Electric fields drop off very quickly away from the source. Generally, around 100 metres (110 yards) from a typical 220,000 volt power line the electric field is unlikely to be high enough to give rise to any adverse health effects, based on our scientific knowledge to date. With 400,000 volt power lines the safe distance is almost double, so at around 200 metres (220 yards) from these lines we would not expect any health problems. This is good news for the estimated 80,000 UK citizens and 250,000 Americans who live close to high voltage (HV) power lines.

Reducing exposure

To protect our health we should limit our exposure to electric fields from power lines as far as possible, but as with all electric fields, it is chronic long-term exposure that is the most damaging. If you pass under power lines while out on a country walk, or while driving, you will only be exposed for a short period. But if your house is within 200 metres (220 yards) of an HV line you may be exposed to the field for most of the day and certainly for all the time you are asleep, when the effects can be most serious (see page 44).

Trees or other buildings between the home and the line may screen you from the electric fields, but this is not always so. A large metal object, such as a corrugated iron barn, would conduct the field so that the end of the metal barn nearest your home could give rise to a locally high electric field.

Using curtains and screens of fine metal mesh at the windows can also screen you from electric fields and several firms sell these (see resources on page 120). But if your house is close to high voltage power lines, the best advice is probably to move home, if you possibly can. If this is not an option, choose to sleep in the rooms farthest away from the power

Case study

Between Aghada and Raffeen in the area of Cork Harbour, there are a number of 220,000 volt power lines, and the fields from these have been found at various distances away. At 10m (11 yards) on either side of the route the electric field is around $4000Vm^{-1}$. At 50m (55 yards) away it has dropped to only $80Vm^{-1}$.

Case study

In 1989 the British Columbia BC Hydro Utility offered to buy the houses of 159 families that lay within 175m (190 yards) of its new 230,000 volt power line, due to concern about electric and magnetic fields. All but six of these families accepted their offer.

Safe distances

The following suggested guidelines for safe distances from power lines err on the side of caution and are based on the US National Council for Radiation Protection assertion that an electric field of $25Vm^{-1}$ does not have adverse side effects.

400,000V	250m (270 yards)
275,000V	200m (220 yards)
132,000V	150m (160 yards)
transformer	25m (27 yards)
substation	100m (110 yards)
cellphone mast	200m (220 yards)

line, and remember that the downstairs rooms will have lower fields than those upstairs, which are nearer the overhead lines.

The human brain adjusts as far as it can to adverse electric fields, but if you go away on vacation it will be unprepared for the effects when you return home. Many people find that they catch a cold soon after returning from a trip away, or that they sleep badly on their first night in a strange place. This suggests that sudden changes in the ambient electric field put stress on the body and immune system. A magnetized mattress may be worth trying – in a study of several types I noted that they seemed to remove some of the damaging perturbations of the electric field (see page 96).

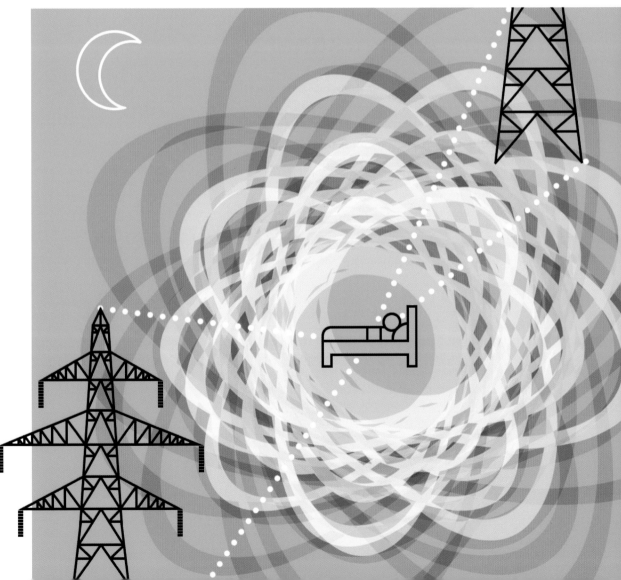

chapter 3
healing with magnets

A wide variety of conflicting theories have been developed to explain how magnets work in healing. Sweeping claims have been made for their healing powers, often based on ancient myth and legend.

Until recently there have been no peer-reviewed scientific studies available to support these claims. But the results from ongoing research in many countries are being published and these back up magnet therapists' claims for the effectiveness of magnets in healing. After a brief look at some of the historical uses of magnets in treating illness, this chapter outlines the mechanisms by which magnets heal, based on scientifically accepted evidence for the physiological effects of magnetic fields.

The next two sections describe treatment plans for specific ailments with static magnets (pages 82–97) and pulsed magnetic fields (pages 100–107), all based on the latest scientific research. The final section explores the wider applications of magnet therapy, including the health benefits of magnetized water, and practical suggestions for treating plants and animals with magnets.

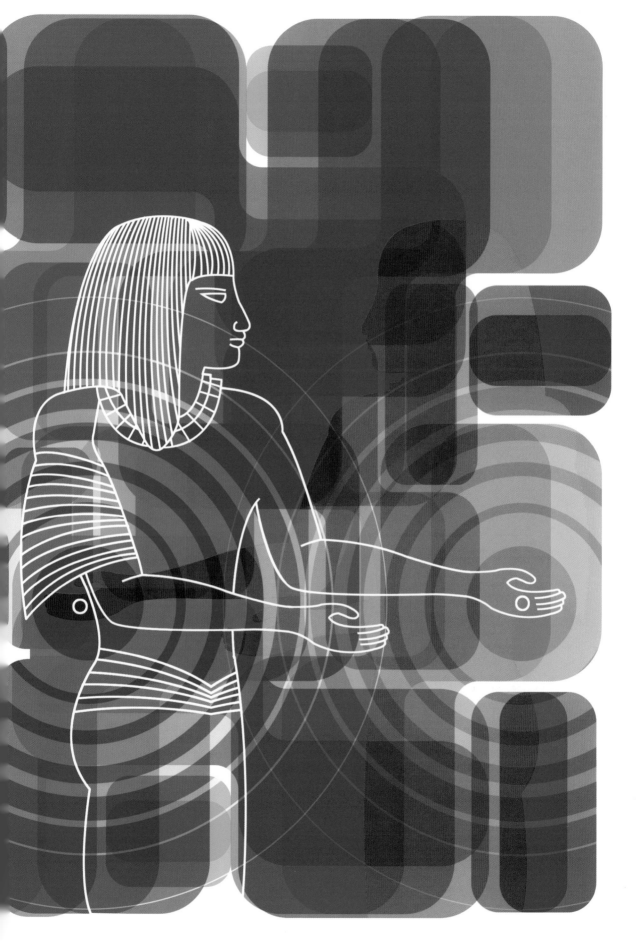

ancient traditions

Magnets have been used in healing for thousands of years.

Healing charges

The Egyptian high priests of Anubis applied cotton "charged with the life of Ptah" for healing. These were cotton cloths that carried either a positive or negative charge and were said to speed the rate of healing. Such cloths probably gained a static electric charge when they were rubbed with another material. This same mechanism is at work when you get a "shock" from a metal part of your car as you get out of it. The shock is the discharge of static electricity – you have become charged with static electricity through friction between your clothing and the car seat.

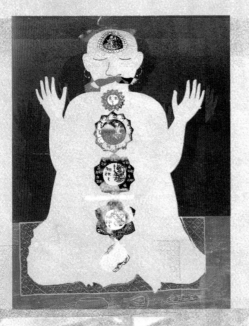

Chinese tradition

The Yellow Emperor's Classic of Internal Medicine, believed to date from the reign of Emperor Huang Ti between 2697 and 2596BC, is the basis of all traditional Chinese medicine. It prescribes placing magnetic stones on specific areas of the body to correct yin and yang imbalances.

Magnetic harmony

The *Vedas*, ancient Hindu scriptures dating from around 1500BC, mention the treatment of disease with ashmana and siktavati, instruments of stone thought to be lodestones. There is also an Indian tradition that the dying should be positioned with their heads toward north, to induce magnetic harmony between Earth and body. In a modern echo of this tradition, many people in India today prefer to sleep in this orientation, which is considered to be the most restful.

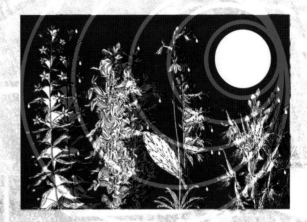

Applying electrical energy

Franz Anton Mesmer, famous for his hypnosis techniques, gained a doctorate from Vienna University in the effects of gravity on health, and in 1775 published a treatise: *On the Medicinal Uses of the Magnet.*

Mesmer believed that we have an electric life force that is disrupted by disease. He argued that by applying external electric fields he could correct the energy disruption and thus cure the disease. At his public clinic for "animal magnetism treatment" in Paris, he would ask women to hold an electrically charged item and stand in a tub of water. Despite the sensationalism of his approach, there is some evidence that it worked.

Prescribing lodestone

The Swiss alchemist and physician Paracelsus (see page 15) used magnets in the treatment of epilepsy, diarrhea, and hemorrhage. He recommended grinding and ingesting lodestone, or collecting dew at the time of the full moon, when there are more positive ions in the atmosphere and the dew would have a positive charge. However, an excess of positive ions is detrimental to health (see page 30).

Preserving youth

An established legend has it that the Egyptian Queen Cleopatra would place a magnetic amulet on her forehead to preserve her youthful looks. This "third eye" area is a pressure point for the pineal gland in many healing traditions, such as shiatsu.

Scientists now recognize that the pineal gland is sensitive to magnetic fields. At night this gland secretes melatonin and sensitizes cell membranes to the reception of repair signals. A magnet placed here could therefore aid the cell repair process and be conducive to deep and refreshing sleep. Even today Tibetan monks place a bar magnet on the forehead to improve concentration and learning ability.

magnet research

The last two centuries have seen increasing interest in the effects of magnetic fields on the body.

In the nineteenth century magnetism was a popular area for research. Eydam wrote about the application of therapeutic magnets in 1843, and Westphal and Gangee reported in 1878 that abnormal skin sensations returned to normal on application of static magnets. In the same year Waldmann's thesis *Der Magnetismus in der Heilkunde* (Magnetism and Health) was probably the first modern treatise on the topic. Benedict, and his contemporary Drozdov, first reported in 1879 that static magnets applied to the body could relieve pain. Benedict coined the word "magnetotherapy" in his work of 1885, and Quinan's *General History of the Application of Magnetism in Medical Science* was published in 1886.

Despite attempts to dismiss magnet therapy as charlatanism, biological scientists' interest in magnetism continued to grow. Medical professionals in the US and Europe were (and often still are) sceptical of the wide claims made for magnets, as they were for other forms of alternative and complementary medicine. For magnets to be sold for therapeutic use, their claims had to be supported by peer-reviewed scientific studies, but getting such studies published in orthodox medical journals was almost impossible.

In the 1960s the Barnothy family set up a laboratory at the College of Pharmacy, University of Illinois, to investigate biological effects of magnetism. In the first of two separate volumes published in that decade, Professor Madeleine Barnothy presented papers from over thirty authors, including a bibliography of the biological effects of static magnetic fields, compiled by Dr Leo Gross of the Waldemar Medical Research Foundation in New York. This listed hundreds of previous studies, some published in the respected periodical *Nature*, indicating that magnet therapy was, at that time, seen as a serious science.

Bioelectromagnetic societies

The First Biomagnetic Symposium was held at the University of Illinois' College of Pharmacy in November 1961. Sixty-five delegates from all over the US attended, and the two-day event included visits to three nearby biomagnetics laboratories. The US Bioelectro-magnetics Society (BEMS) was not formed until 19 years later. In 1998 this 700-strong society was accorded educational status by the US medical establishment. It now organizes sponsored conferences and has a web-based forum for the exchange of ideas worldwide.

The European Bioelectromagnetics Association is younger and smaller with about 290 members. Its biennial congresses attract more Eastern bloc participants and thus present science not reported at the BEMS meetings. The International Commission on Non-Ionizing Radiation also holds occasional symposia, and publishes the proceedings.

Research worldwide

After World War II the Eastern bloc countries were very keen to develop inexpensive methods of cure, to avoid reliance on expensive drugs manufactured in the west. At the 1996 World Congress on Magnetotherapy in London, delegates from the former Soviet Union reported on magnet treatments with static magnets and alternating devices. In the Czech Republic Dr Jiri Jerabek has compiled a list of hundreds of clinical studies of magnet therapy. Similarly in the Ukraine there is an established body of clinical evidence of the efficacy of magnet therapy, and one expert, Dr Sergei Gerasimov, reports trials on children with asthma using magnets and also radio waves.

The Japanese also have a long history of magnet therapy research and practice, building on their tradition of using non-chemical methods of healing, such as shiatsu. In 1976 the scientist Nakagawa undertook a major review of over 100 studies on magnets dating back to the 1950s. In his view magnetic fields redress the imbalance caused by the weakening geomagnetic field and the advent of artificial alternating electric and magnetic fields. The development of lightweight powerful neodymium magnets in Japan in 1983 triggered more research into their therapeutic uses, since they make it possible to apply a strong local magnetic field with a very small magnet. The Japanese firm Nikken, now one of the largest companies in the world, manufactures and sells magnets and magnetic appliances such as insoles, knee pads, and mattress pads worldwide.

A twenty first century therapy

More recently the failure of conventional western medicine to develop satisfactory drug treatments for degenerative and immune system diseases have led to increased interest in many forms of complementary therapy, and magnet therapy in particular. There are ongoing research projects at several universities, including the Vanderbilt University, Nashville, Tennessee, which held a World Congress in 1999. In the UK, the Royal Society of Medicine's sports medicine department is now taking an interest in magnet treatments. The advertisement regulatory authorities have also helped the science, by insisting on clinical trials proving the efficacy of any products advertised. In consequence the number of good quality peer-reviewed studies is increasing, and with it greater medical acceptance of the role of magnets in healing.

areas of magnet research

Evidence shows that magnets may have a role to play in treating a variety of conditions.

Applications for magnets are still being discovered, and more research into their efficacy is being carried out as magnet manufacturers seek to justify their claims for the products they sell. The following is just some of the research showing promising results.

Cancer treatment

The 1960s saw the first research into the use of magnets in treating cancer in animals. This found that static magnets appeared to reduce solid tumors. In a study in 1964, Vernon Reno and Leo Nutini from the Institute of Divi Thomae, Cincinnati, Ohio exposed the cancer cells of Sarcoma 37 tumors to various field strengths between 80 and 7300 gauss. They found that with the highest field level, the uptake of oxygen in the cancer cells was reduced by 50 per cent. It seems likely that this lowered the cells' already improverished adenosine triphosphate (ATP) synthesis, so that some cells did not survive. This reduced oxygen intake contrasts with the increased oxygen intake in normal cells under static magnet influence (see below) and seems to confirm the views of 1931 Nobel prizewinner Otto Warburg, that cancer arises from a metabolic change leading to faulty cell respiration. His explanation (see right) has been refined by further research at Coghill Research Laboratories.

Bone fractures

Art Pilla and the late Andy Bassett, working in Columbia University, New York in the 1970s, developed the use of pulsed electromagnetic fields to repair non-union bone fractures – where the two parts of a broken bone refuse to knit together. The electromagnetic fields they applied to the fracture mimicked the body's own endogenous fields and

Metabolic changes in cancer

In normal cell respiration, oxygen is vital for the synthesis of the energy molecule ATP (see page 71). But if the electron transport pathway is blocked (and most carcinogens can do this) ATP is not synthesized. In such cases cells revert to a less efficient way of making ATP, called glycolysis, which does not require oxygen.

Glycolysis requires large amounts of glucose, so the cell either stops making the glycoproteins on its plasma membrane surfaces, or it starts resorbing them to obtain its vital sugar. But most of these glycoproteins are the cell's means of information reception. Without them the cell is "blind" to regulatory growth control signals from the brain, so it divides out of control and no longer responds to contact inhibition (where it stops dividing when in contact with other cells of the same body). All these signs are seen in cancer cells.

stimulated repair. The US Federal Drug Administration (FDA) has approved at least one such device, but it may only be used for non-unions – where the bone has refused to join sometimes for several years – and not for fresh fractures. According to Dr Pilla, his approach has saved some 10,000 patients from amputation over the years.

The ElectroBiology devices (EBI) that emerged from this research are widely used in the US today, and the approach is being studied in British hospitals.

Pain relief

As early as 1938, Scandinavian Karen M Hansen reported that static magnets alleviated disorders such as sciatica, lumbago, and joint pain. Her 1944 paper in the medical journal *Acta Medica Scandinavica* aimed to prove objectively that magnets influence the human body. Measuring air intake and output in a total of 130 people with normal metabolism, and a similar number of controls, she showed that oxygen absorption increased when a magnet was placed 3cm (1.2in) from the left temple. The field strength was not stated. Increased oxygen absorption makes more oxygen available in the blood, which in turn helps muscles to work more efficiently and therefore reduces muscular pain. This mechanism is explained in more detail on pages 76–7.

In a more recent trial in 1998 at Vanderbilt University, Nashville, Tennessee a painful stimulant derived from peppers was injected under volunteers' skin. All the volunteers found that the four neodymium magnets applied reduced the subsequent pain levels significantly.

Reduction in pain was among the benefits reported by Sasa Moslavac, whose team worked at the war rehabilitation centre at Varazdinske, Toplice, treating victims of the 1992 Croatian war. Between 1992 and 1995 they used static magnets on over 1200 patients, mostly suffering war wounds and fractures with subsequently low mobility. According to their records, over 88 per cent of their cases refused to interrupt the magnetic field treatment because it was so effective in reducing pain and improving limb mobility.

how cells make energy

All the body's functions depend on chemical reactions in the cells.

We all think of ourselves as individuals, but in reality each of us is only collections of billions of microscopic cells about ten millionths of a metre across. These cells have internal components called organelles to maintain their normal business of taking in and organizing nutrients, and expelling the waste products of metabolism. Nearly 90 per cent of the energy we use to run our bodies comes from organelles called mitochondria. One cell alone might have several hundred of these mitochondria inside it, particularly the brain and muscle cells. Indeed if we take away the 70 per cent of us which is water, nearly half the remaining dry tissue is mitochondria.

These important cell components have their own separate DNA, and some scientists believe that they were at some past stage in evolution separate creatures, imported into our cells because they can make energy much more efficiently than the cells themselves. This energy is in the form of the adenosine triphosphate (ATP) molecule, which is the universal energy molecule of living creatures.

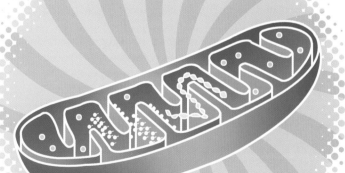

Mitochondrion
The mitochondria are the powerhouses of the cell, making energy available through a series of chemical reactions.

Cell respiration

This means the process by which cells make energy, through a series of chemical reactions.

Oxygen breathed into the lungs passes into the blood, combining with the hemoglobin (iron) molecules in the red blood cells. This oxygen-rich blood is then transported to the body tissues and passes into the cell.

The mitochondria separate hydrogen atoms from their electrons and create an electrical potential difference across their inner membranes. By this process they develop enough energy to weld a third phosphate on to adenosine diphosphate (ADP) to make adenosine triphosphate (ATP). This process (chemio-osmosis) is how most of our energy is made.

The oxygen molecules are there to "catch" any electrons left over at the end of the process, acting as a final electron acceptor.

The role of enzymes

The speed of the cell respiration process depends on specific enzymes in the cell, which control the speed of the chemical reactions. The respiratory enzymes control the respiration process rigorously, so that excess electrons do not escape to damage other cells by free radical action. When there is no need for ATP the enzymes slow the reaction and put the cell "into neutral".

Where the ATP is used

Once synthesized by the mitochondria, ATP circulates in the body fluids and can be used by any other cell to which it is made available. It is used for a variety of purposes, from the effort of cell division (mitosis) or protein forming (synthesis) to the movement of muscles. Even thinking and breathing requires energy.

enzyme reactions

Magnets affect the rate of enzyme reactions, and thus the chemical reactions important for life processes.

Enzymes are proteins that act as catalysts, either speeding up or slowing down reactions. By selectively lowering the energy needed for chemical reactions, enzymes can determine the speed and course of the reactions very specifically. Magnetic fields appear to affect this electron-related process: the field causes electrons to spin uniformly and in the same direction (see page 21) and thus affects reactions. Several studies have shown that the effect of the magnetic field is actually bi-phasic: when the reaction is going too fast it slows it down, but when it is going too slowly it speeds it up. The enzyme experiments described below show how a weak magnetic field, as low as 60 gauss (6mT), can have a physiological effect.

Magnets can speed reactions

In the 1960s, Dr George Akoyunoglou, a post-doctoral research fellow of the US National Academy of Sciences, demonstrated that magnetic fields can speed up enzyme activity. In more than twenty experiments he exposed the plant enzyme carboxydismutase, prepared from spinach chloroplasts, to a static magnetic field of 20,000 gauss (2 tesla) – the same sort of field strength as used in an MRI scanner. His results, which were published in 1964 in the respected journal *Nature*, showed a profound activating effect of 14–20 per cent on the enzyme. With restrained excitement he concluded, "The activating effect of a magnetic field is quite a new discovery, and opens up a fascinating field for new studies".

A more recent joint study from Bulgaria and New York's Mount Sinai Hospital (Gemishev, Tsoloova et al, 1994) found statistically significant effects on respiratory enzymes in wheat seedlings using magnetic field strengths between 60 and 2000 gauss (6 and 200mT) and exposure periods between six and twenty five hours. In this study there was a 94 per cent increase in an important respiratory enzyme, succinate oxidase, in only sixty minutes.

Magnets can slow reactions down

When electrons leave an atom for some reason, such as friction or attraction from another atom, for a moment they are free to travel. These electrons are called free radicals and each seeks to find another electron and make a pair spinning antiparallel (each spinning in opposite directions). This process of pairing is known as radical pair formation. During this brief moment of freedom a magnetic field acting on the electron may cause it to change direction. The result is to increase the period of time taken for radical pair formation and therefore to complete the reaction process.

Two scientists from the University of Utah, Tim Harkins and Charles Grissom, set up an experiment to see if a magnetic field could affect enzymes in this way. They placed a mixture of enzyme and substrate (the substance on which the enzyme acts) in a clear glass flask with the poles of an electromagnet on either side. The mixture became cloudy when the enzyme was active, so measuring the extent of the cloudiness using a spectrophotometer gave a measure of enzyme activity. In the experiment the electromagnet was switched on for a period and the effect of the magnetic field on the enzyme activity assessed.

The scientists found that the mixture became cloudy up to 25 per cent more slowly when the magnetic field was switched on. By varying the strength of the field they also discovered that the strongest field is not necessarily the most effective: the slowdown began at 500 gauss and peaked at 1500, after which it began to fall again. Thus the correct field strength is necessary for optimal effect.

improving circulation

A magnetic field speeds blood flow and reduces blockage in veins and arteries.

Just under one per cent of our blood is charged particles or ions. These include sodium (Na^+) and chlorine (Cl^-) which together make salt, thus explaining why blood tastes salty.

Suppose that a number of ions are moving in the blood within an artery. If we place the artery between the poles of a static magnet the ions are now moving within a magnetic field. They then polarize, the negatively charged ones moving in the opposite direction to the positive, so drifting to opposite sides of the artery. This polarization in turn produces an electric field, and its minute potential difference leads to a small induced current flow. Any ions that have become attached to the artery walls can be freed by this current to flow back into the main stream.

This same action is also observed in water pipes "furred up" with limescale: not only are the salts kept in solution by a static magnet applied outside the pipe, but any existing blockage in the pipes is gradually descaled. The technique has been commonly used for many years in industry, and works just as well for veins and arteries blocked with unwanted obstacles to circulation.

In the artery the flow velocity is directly proportional to the voltage that builds up across the artery, and this in turn is dependent on the magnetic field strength applied. In cases of severe blockage there is a potential danger that the application of very strong magnets could rapidly speed the blood flow. This could then shift the deposited materials, still grouped together, to another part of the circulation system, leading to a blockage elsewhere. In such cases the best field strengths are not necessarily the strongest. The maximum that should be applied initially is around 950 gauss, though as improvement proceeds this strength can be increased.

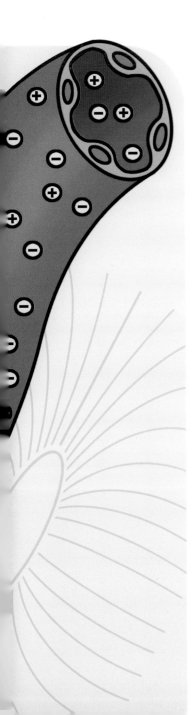

Treating gout with magnets

One of the earliest recorded therapeutic uses of magnets for circulation problems is in treating gout. It is said that Cleopatra used magnets to treat her Roman lovers. Gout arises from the build-up in the bloodstream of uric acid crystals, to the point where they restrict blood flow. This is particularly noticeable where the blood vessel passes over the bone of the big toe, leading to such acute pain that the sufferer can hardly bear the toe to be touched. The uric acid crystals can originally arise from drinking excessive alcohol, but gout also affects elderly people who hardly drink, and the problem can become chronic. Conventional treatment is usually by means of non-steroidal anti-inflammatory drugs (NSAIDs) but these can take several days to have an effect and eventually they become ineffective resulting in the need for stronger steroidal treatment. Long-term use of NSAIDs may also cause damage to the internal organs.

Using a magnet of at least 950 gauss applied to the blood vessel usually brings relief in minutes and there are no side effects. The magnet can be placed inside a sock, with a second magnet on the outside to hold it in position near the painful area.

Treating swelling with magnets

Another common circulatory problem is swelling or edema in the leg. This occurs where the tissue under the skin becomes swollen by fluids and is unable to escape. The condition is commonly seen in the elderly, particularly bedridden patients, and is also common in the obese. An associated problem is crural ulcers of the leg, where in severe edema cases the skin begins to break, leading to wounds that can prove extremely difficult to heal.

Applying a 950 gauss magnet to the skin directly over the bandaged ulcer improves the blood circulation in the area so that excess fluid can be transported away from it via the bloodstream. For edema only, the magnet should be applied over the swelling, or to the wrist or ankle for a more general but slower effect. The magnets can be held in place in an elastic stocking or a bandage, with another magnet on the outside to anchor it. Ensure that the bandages are not so tight that they further restrict the circulation you are trying to improve. Treatment for hourly periods over about three weeks should show an improvement.

pain relief

Recent research points to some ways in which magnets can relieve pain.

Carlton Hazlewood has been investigating the effects of magnetic fields on pain relief for years at the Department of Molecular Physiology and Biophysics at Baylor College of Medicine, Houston, Texas. His 1997 double-blind pilot study of response to static magnetic fields in patients recovering from polio, showed a clearly positive effect. It was published in a reputable peer-reviewed journal, but nevertheless came in for some criticism because all the patients, whether using magnetic fields or placebo, reported some improvement.

The same year Hazlewood presented a fascinating paper at the annual International Conference on Stress in Montreux. He proposed that T-lymphocytes, the white blood cells that protect us from infection, play an important role in pain relief. According to his theory, it is the distribution of T-lymphocytes in the various phases of their cell cycle that is responsible for the degree of chronic pain suffered. When a noxious agent is detected in the body, the T-lymphocytes prepare for battle by entering the first phase of the cycle, which is the pain-causing phase. In Hazlewood's study, relief of chronic pain was associated with an almost synchronous shift of the T-lymphocytes into their next phase, the synthesis phase.

This suggests that applying a static magnetic field reduces the pain sensation, by helping the T-lymphocytes to shift to their synthesis phase.

The effect of magnets on endorphins

At the same ground-breaking conference, Saul Liss, a consultant from Paterson, New Jersey, reported a simple experiment to study the effect of a static magnetic field on beta endorphins – the body's natural painkillers. He exposed his subjects' palms for fifteen minutes to a 3950 gauss (395mT) static magnet and measured the effect by taking 15ml (0.5fl oz) blood samples

Case study

In his 1976 review of 68 research reports and books, Dr Kyoichi Nakagawa, director of the Isuzu Hospital, Tokyo, found seven separate studies reporting relief of shoulder pain and stiffness in patients wearing magnetic bracelets. Those wearing the real magnets, of strengths between 200 and 1300 gauss, reported typical improvements of 78 per cent compared with only 17 per cent in the controls group who wore dummy magnets.

One of these reports found that the 1300 gauss magnets were more effective than the weaker 200 gauss versions (Yamada et al, 1976, unpublished report to Japanese Health Ministry). From his own experience and the available evidence, Nakagawa concluded that static fields needed to be at least 500 gauss to be effective.

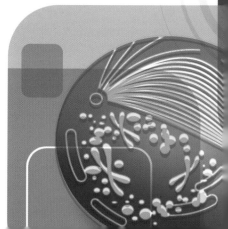

from the forearm vein at the start of the experiment, then at 60 minutes, and at 130 minutes after exposure to the magnet.

Liss found that the number of beta endorphins in the blood were increased by 25 per cent 60 minutes after exposure, and by 45 per cent 130 minutes after exposure.

The connection between rising endorphin levels and shifting T-lymphocyte cell cycles is not difficult to make. Both of these are activated by wounds, which give out an electric current of injury during the healing process. In response to this current, the level of pain-killing beta endorphins in the blood increases, and the T-lymphocytes are urgently attracted to the wound site to protect the body against pathogens that could enter the wound.

the power of magnetic bracelets

Bracelets containing high strength magnets can reduce muscle or joint pain anywhere in the body.

Several manufacturers produce magnetic bracelets to be worn around the wrist. Tests have shown that provided the magnetic strength is at least 500 gauss, they can effectively reduce joint pain far from the wrist such as arthritic pain in the knee joints. Why is this?

The blood permeates the body, carrying with it energy-giving oxygen, the cellular and fluid components of the immune system, taking away waste gases such as carbon dioxide, and acting as a coolant or a heater depending on the need.

Apart from the saline solution that comprises about half of it, blood is composed of white and red cells and platelets. The platelets are there to assist in coagulation, and they do this as a result of their electric charges – oppositely charged platelets are attracted to each other and clump together. Red blood cells are negatively charged and are repelled by the walls of the arteries and veins, also negatively charged. This repulsive force helps them flow freely through the body. Provided it is strong enough, a static magnetic field speeds and improves the blood flow, as we saw on pages 74–5.

Each red blood cell contains millions of hemoglobin molecules, each with a central iron atom that is affected by magnetic fields. Through a subtle method, which is still not fully understood but probably developed through evolution in the Earth's magnetic field, a static magnetic field helps hemoglobin carry out its task of carrying oxygen to the muscle tissues. Once there, the oxygen fulfils its role as an electron acceptor in the final part of energy synthesis (see page 71). So by improving the ability of hemoglobin molecules to carry oxygen, a magnetic field helps muscles to gain energy. With this extra energy, the muscles can work for longer before they become tired and start to ache.

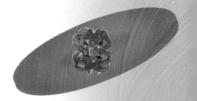

Relieving joint pain

As we age joint pain is common, because our joints wear out with use (osteoarthritis). As the surfaces in the joints deteriorate, the bones start to rub together. This generates electric fields, just as friction between your hair and a comb can generate a static electric field. My own research work with the body's endogenous fields convinces me that any unusual electric fields signal to the white blood cells that something foreign and possibly noxious is nearby, stimulating them into battle action. As Carlton Hazlewood has found, applying a static magnetic field can shift the white blood cells into the next phase of their cell cycle, which is accompanied by a dramatic reduction in pain (see page 76).

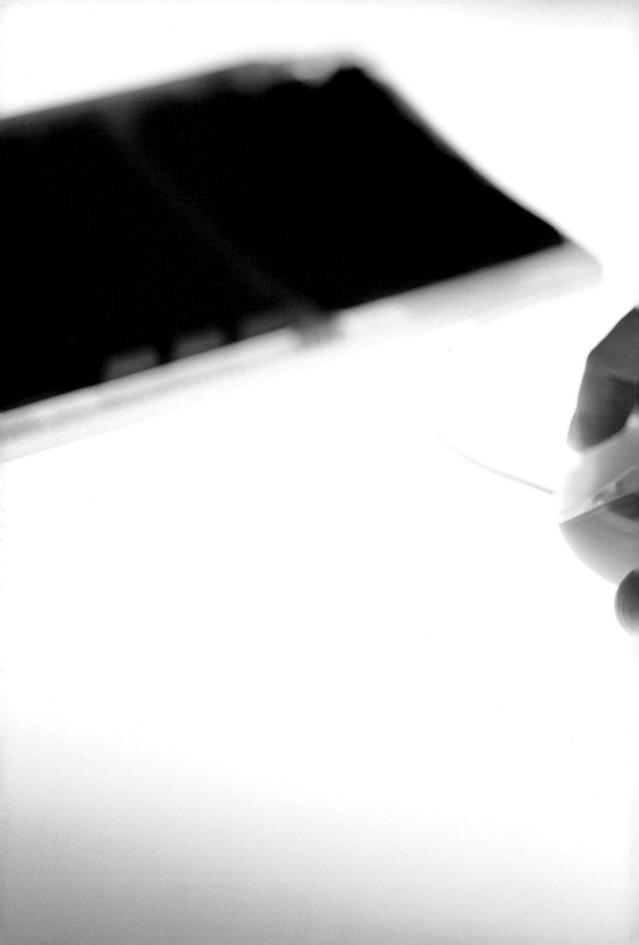

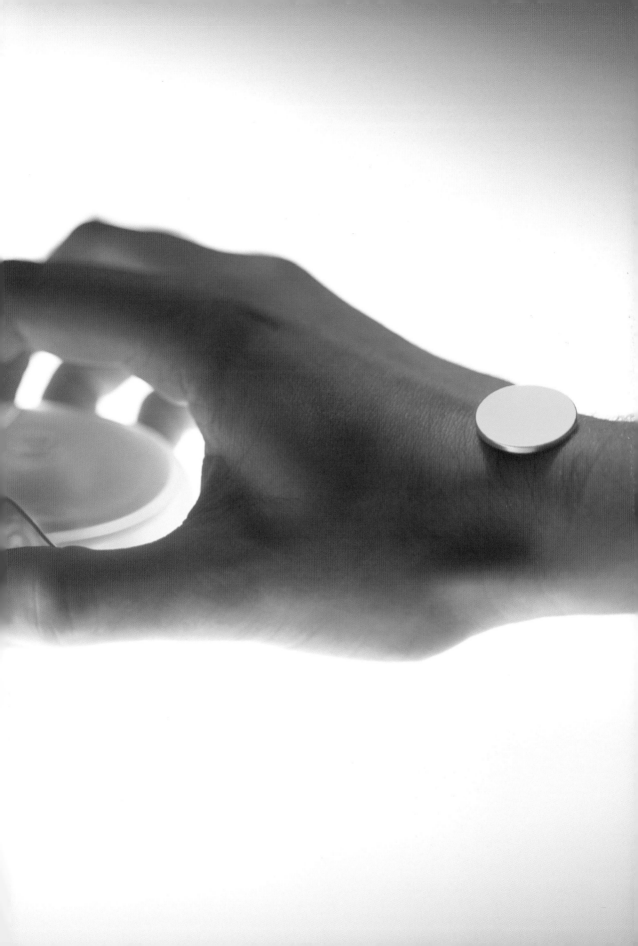

magnet treatments

Guidance for using magnets to treat common ailments.

The treatment plans on pages 86–97 give clear guidance and instructions for treating a range of common conditions that typically respond well to magnet therapy. Before trying the treatments, read the notes on safety and when not to use magnets, below. The strength of magnet to use is given in each treatment, but pages 84–5 provide some general guidance on the different types of magnet available and techniques for applying them to the body.

Safety of magnetic fields

The UK National Radiation Protection Board (NRPB) have investigated the safety of exposure to powerful static magnetic fields and have not found any evidence of harmful effects from fields up to 2 tesla. That is just as well really, because the MRI (magnetic resonance imaging) technology used in hospitals for body and brain scans apply fields of up to 4 tesla. In their recommendations for safe exposure the NRPB have divided 2 tesla by ten to obtain a value of 200mT (or 2000 gauss). This is the upper limit they recommend for exposure over any twenty four hour period. The treatments on pages 86–97 all use magnets below this strength.

Magnet therapy practitioners usually recommend that once the magnet has done its job it should be removed, allowing the body to heal itself naturally.

Combining magnet therapy with other techniques

Magnet treatments can safely be used in conjunction with other medical and complementary techniques, and may indeed enhance their effectiveness. A magnetic field speeds up or slows down chemical reactions in the body to their optimum rate (see page 72) and a stabilizing effect will also be seen in any reactions at a cellular level induced by therapies such as acupuncture, or reflexology, or by medicinal drugs. In fact magnets have been shown to enhance conventional drug treatments in this way so that the dose needed is reduced, sometimes to one tenth of the previous requirement. It is not possible to say with accuracy what the effects are with any specific medication, because the research simply hasn't been done yet.

Always consult your doctor or medical practitioner before using magnet treatments, and do not reduce the dosage of prescribed medication without medical guidance.

Contraindications for magnet treatment

Very little research has been published on the effects of static magnetic fields in specific conditions. Until such evidence is available it is wise to err on the side of caution. Observe any advice or contraindications supplied with your magnets and do not treat anyone with any of the following conditions.

Research

The number of hooks on the sperm heads of rats was reduced after exposure to a 7000 gauss static field for 35 days, suggesting lowered potency (Tablado, Perez-Sanchez et al. 1998).

Mice exposed from birth to a 4200 gauss static magnet grew significantly less in the first 11 days than mice exposed to a dummy magnet (Barnothy, 1963). However another study found no differences in rats or mice after four weeks' exposure to a range of field strengths (Bellosi, Sutter-Dub et al. 1984).

A study using chick embryos found that after 13 days' exposure to a static magnetic field the cerebellum cells showed signs of degeneration and delay in the process of neuronal differentiation (Espinar, Piera et al. 1997).

• **Pregnant women and infants under three months**

There is no study proving adverse effects of static magnets in pregnancy on the mother or unborn child, and such a study would not be approved by an ethical committee. However there are several studies reporting adverse effects on animal young, embryos, and sperm (see left).

• **Hemophilia and bleeding**

Since one effect of a magnetic field is to increase blood flow, there could be unwanted side effects from magnet treatment. For the same reason do not use magnets on anyone who has recently had surgery.

• **Metal implants**

Any metal in the body will concentrate magnetic fields unpredictably, which may be counterproductive to the treatment.

• **Pacemakers**

Magnetic fields can affect the heartbeat, so pacemaker wearers should not use magnets.

If you suffer any adverse effects after using magnets, report these to the magnet manufacturer. Most keep records of such reports and will be keen to warn other purchasers of any contraindications for use.

which magnet to use

There are a number of factors to consider when buying magnets for home treatment.

Many devices on the market involve applying static magnets to the body: bracelets, pendants, insoles for shoes, magnets incorporated in clothing and belts, magnets in seats and seat covers, and magnets in mattresses. Often these devices are supplied without any details of the strengths of the magnets in them, but a reputable supplier should be able to give you this information. Also their use can be fairly restricted – you cannot easily apply a magnet bracelet to an aching back.

Magnets that can be placed anywhere on the body are clearly more versatile for treatment. And if you can only apply one field strength with your magnet its use may be limited, since different conditions require different magnetic field strengths for treatment.

Coghill Research Laboratories produce neodymium magnets (see page 23) in sets of two, to be used with or without a spacer between them to deliver a range of field strengths. Used together without spacers the two magnets create a very powerful field, typically around 2000 gauss. When the spacer is inserted between the magnets the field becomes much lower (1450 gauss), while one magnet used alone gives a field strength of around 700 gauss. Any set of magnets and spacers should be supplied with details of the field strengths possible and clear instructions on how to combine the magnets and spacers to achieve these strengths.

Applying the magnets

The treatment plans on pages 86–97 explain clearly where to apply the magnets. One of the easiest ways to apply a magnet to the body is to hold it in place in your clothing with another magnet, or a magnetic coin, on the other side to stop it sliding. If this is not practical, you can attach it with sticking plaster or microporous tape, or hold it in place with a bandage.

North and south poles

Some magnet therapy practitioners maintain that there is a therapeutic difference in whether the north or south pole is applied nearest the body. I have yet to find a single peer-reviewed study supporting this notion and I expect that most physicists would also be astonished if such differences existed.

All magnets have a north and south pole, so named because one pole always points toward the Earth's magnetic north. The magnetic field flowing out from one pole curls around the magnet to arrive at the other pole. So putting the north pole of a magnet on your body means that its north pole influence (underneath the magnet) is balanced by its south pole influence, perhaps only 3mm ($\frac{1}{8}$in) away. Thus the effect will be the same, whichever pole you apply.

Caution

Always observe the notes on safety on page 82 and the contraindications for treatment listed on page 83.

Types of magnet

Some manufacturers and therapists describe their magnets as unipolar. This does not mean that these magnets have only one pole. Such a magnet does not exist: however thinly the magnet is sliced, one end will always be the north pole and one the south. What therapists mean by unipolar is that only one pole is applied to the body.

A bipolar magnet applies both poles simultaneously. A horsehoe magnet is an example, though these are not used for therapy. However some magnetic bracelets and other devices contain magnets arranged in a bipolar array, with their opposite poles adjacent to each other. The manufacturers claim that this increases the gradient of the magnetic flux within the body, giving a stronger therapeutic effect. However, the field strength is much less than with a unipolar magnet, because the opposite poles tend to cancel each other out.

Following the treatment plans

The treatment plans on pages 86–97 give clear guidance on the strength of magnet and how many magnets to use, how often to apply them, and for how long each time. This information is based on the findings on optimal exposures for different conditions from a large number of clinical trials undertaken worldwide.

The magnetic strengths given in the treatment plans are the strengths in gauss "at the pole face", meaning on the pole of the magnet, where it touches the skin. Some effects are best achieved by using quite small field strengths, not necessarily the highest available. Before following the treatment plans make sure that you know the field strength at the pole face of your magnets.

Devising your own treatments

Once you have had some experience of using magnets and are familiar with their applications outlined in this book, you may like to experiment a little. Static magnets with field strengths up to 2000 gauss are very safe to use, so you are unlikely to do any harm provided you follow the safety advice and contraindications given on pages 82–3.

For the length and frequency of treatment, as a rule of thumb, remove your magnet when you start to feel better. But put it back on again if the pain returns. As a general guide, do not apply magnets for more than eight hours at a time.

muscle and joint pain

- lower back pain
- tennis elbow and frozen shoulder
- upper limb disorders

People sit down too much these days: we drive for long distances, sit all day in offices, and watch TV most evenings. As a result our blood circulation becomes more sluggish, which means that less oxygen is delivered by our hemoglobin to muscular tissues.

Muscles still need energy, if only to hold the skeletal frame in the correct posture, and one result of poor circulation is muscle pain, especially in the lower back. Applying static magnets can relieve muscle and joint pain, and the results are sometimes spectacularly immediate.

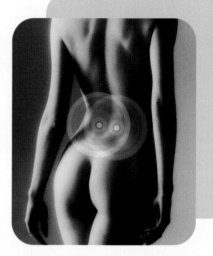

Lower back pain
Magnets to use: two minimum 950 gauss, up to a maximum 2000 gauss

Feel down either side of your spine until you reach your pelvis. Place magnets about 2.5cm (1in) above this point and about 5cm (2in) on either side of the spine. You will probably feel that these areas are the seat of the ache anyway. Keep the magnets in position by placing a small coin on the other side of your clothing. Apply the magnets for about 30 minutes, but it does no harm to leave them there overnight.

Tennis elbow and frozen shoulder
Magnets to use: one 2000 gauss

These nagging chronic conditions (including chronic tendonitis) are somewhat stubborn, but relief can be surprisingly sudden. Place a 2000 gauss magnet where you feel the pain, held in place with a small iron-rich coin on the other side of your clothing. You should feel an improvement after about 30 minutes, but you can safely leave the magnet on overnight.

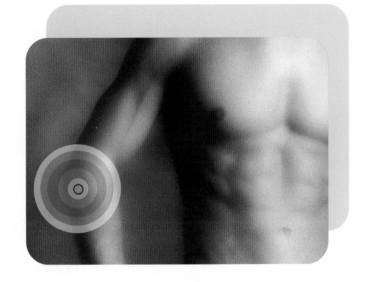

Upper limb disorders
Magnets to use: two 2000 gauss

This covers carpal tunnel syndrome, tenosynovitis, and repetitive strain injury (RSI). Apply two 2000 gauss magnets, one either side of the wrist where you feel the pain. Hold them in place with a glove and leave them on overnight. These problems became common in the 1980s among computer operators, but since the introduction of low radiation screens the incidence has decreased, suggesting that the conditions are radiation related.

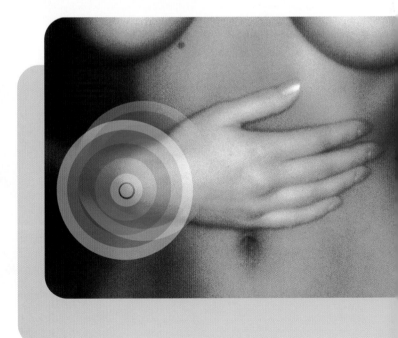

• arthritis and rheumatism

Rheumatism is a general term describing aches and pains in bones, muscles, joints, and tissues, and so includes arthritis, which affects the joints. Osteoarthritis is a degenerative disease, caused by wear and tear on the joints through use, particularly in the hands and knees. Over the age of sixty, everyone will show some form of arthritis in X-rays, even if they do not suffer the symptoms.

Since the degenerative changes are irreversible, there is no cure for arthritis and medical treatment is with non-steroidal anti-inflammatory drugs (NSAIDs). Magnets can dramatically reduce the pain of rheumatic and arthritic complaints even when the sufferer has had many years of discomfort. Do not be tempted to leave the magnets on after the pain is reduced, since the alleviative effect of the magnetic field is reduced if you are exposed to it constantly.

Pain relief
Magnets to use: one 2000 gauss

Apply a magnet where you feel the pain, held in place by a coin on the opposite side of your clothing. Leave it in place until the pain subsides. About 10 minutes is usually sufficient. Once the pain is reduced, remove the magnet.

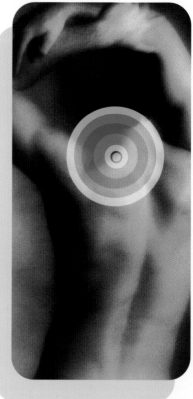

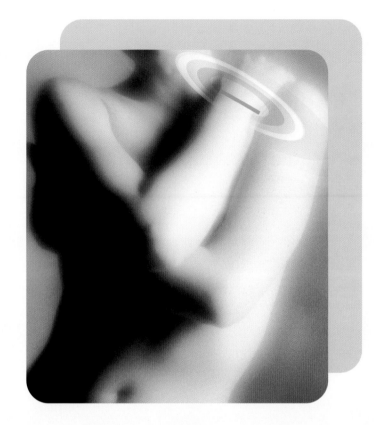

Magnetic bracelets

Bracelets containing magnets can be very effective in relieving rheumatic or arthritic pain anywhere in the body (see page 78). Choose a bracelet with a minimum strength of 500 gauss to wear continually. Bracelets with stronger magnets – around 2000 gauss – should only be worn at night. Ensure the bracelet is close fitting so that the magnets are as near as possible to your wrist.

Copper bracelets

Arthritic and rheumatic pain tend to be greater when there is a high level of positive ions in the air (for example, before a thunderstorm) and reduce when there are more negative ions. Since copper ions are positively charged, a copper bracelet attracts beneficial negatively charged ions to your body. You should wash the bracelet daily under running water, to remove the build-up of free electrons so that it can function properly.

Research

There is much anecdotal evidence on the effectiveness of magnets in treating rheumatism and arthritis, but few clinical trials have been carried out. In his 1996 literature review Dr Jiri Jerabek, of the Czech Republic's National Institute for Health, quotes an early study of rheumatoid arthritis (Aryshenkskaya, 1977) where patients applied 150–400 gauss magnets for 10 minutes and for 10–20 exposures. They responded well in the early stages, but there was sometimes an initial impairment followed by a variable improvement.

respiratory problems
- coughs
- asthma

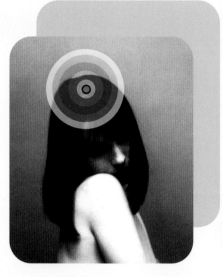

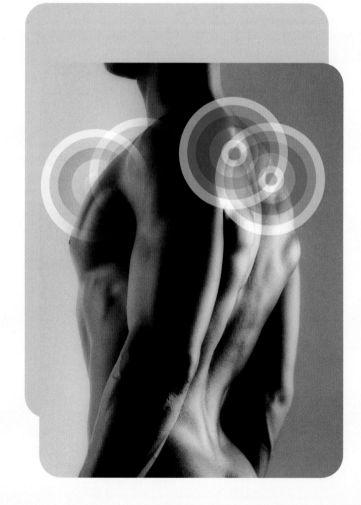

Coughs
Magnets to use: two 950 gauss

Apply two magnets on the chest and two on the back for 25 minutes daily, for 10–15 days. If the cough clears within this period, stop the treatment. For bronchitis, apply the magnet to the middle of the top of the head for 25 minutes daily, for 10–15 days. Use this treatment in conjunction with your usual medication and inform your doctor that you are using magnets as well.

Asthma
Magnets to use: four 2000 gauss

One in seven children in Britain is likely to suffer from asthma at some time, a horrendous statistic, paralleled in the US and Australia. Continue with the prescribed treatment, and let your doctor know that you will be using magnet treatment as well.

The conventional treatment is to place 2000 gauss magnets over the chest and back, over the bronchial tubes.

Magnet therapist and medical doctor Michael Tierra places 3000 gauss magnets 2cm (1in) either side of the spine, level with the space between the seventh cervical and first thoracic vertebrae. (The seventh cervical vertebra is the most prominent bone at the base of your neck when you lean your head forward.) These points are acupuncture points used to treat asthma in traditional Chinese medicine.

For each treatment, apply the magnets for around one hour daily, for a period of 20–30 days. You can also apply the magnets during an asthma attack, but only after you have taken the appropriate emergency action.

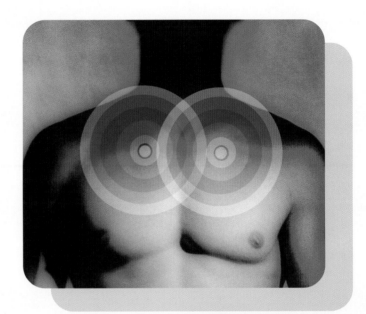

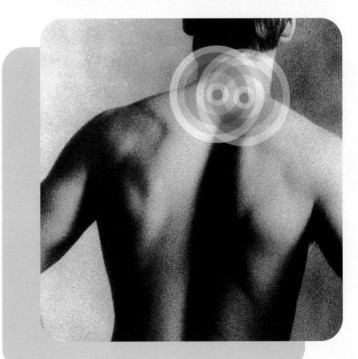

- **constipation**
- **menstrual cramps**

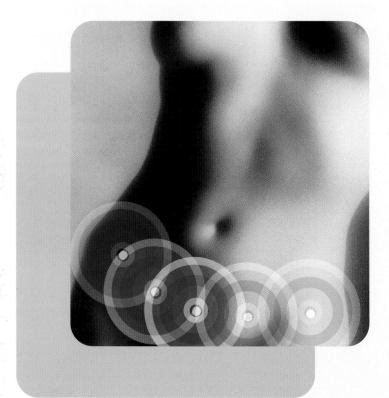

Constipation
Magnets to use: five 950 gauss

Clinical studies have tended to concentrate on inflammatory intestinal conditions rather than on constipation, but personal testimonies recommend magnet treatment. Apply the five magnets in a horizontal row across the lower abdomen, for no longer than three hours. Their effect may be quite sudden, so be warned!

Case study
My wife became constipated after giving birth to our son. Anxious to avoid taking any medicines that could be passed on to the baby through breast milk, she applied magnets across her lower abdomen when she went to bed. The next morning I was happy to hear that the problem had been solved successfully during the night.

Menstrual cramps
Magnets to use: one 400 gauss

Magnets relieve cramp by improving
blood circulation to the area. Apply a
400 gauss magnet to the abdomen,
midway between the navel and the
pubic bone, for up to 10 minutes. The
cramp should ease in this time. It is
best to be cautious when applying
magnets near the reproductive system,
and to use them for the minimum time
necessary whenever the cramps occur.

Research
The relief from menstrual cramps was
only one of the benefits reported by
Suprun and Kerkhevitsch, working in
St Petersburg, in their 1989 review of
gynecological studies. In one trial
women with bad period pains
benefited from applying a 400 gauss
magnet to the abdomen during the
second half of the menstrual cycle, for
30 minutes daily. After three series
with a one-month interval between
treatments, over 90 per cent of the
patients reported an improvement.

Other successful magnet treatments
were for treating thrush, lactostasis,
exocervical erosions, endocervitis, and
restoration of conceptual capability.
Most of these studies were carried out
in Moscow and St Petersburg, and
except for abstracts, are available only
in Russian.

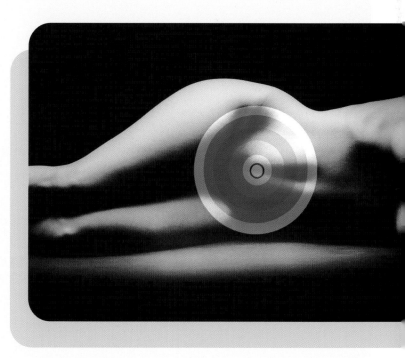

- inflammation
- headaches
- jet lag

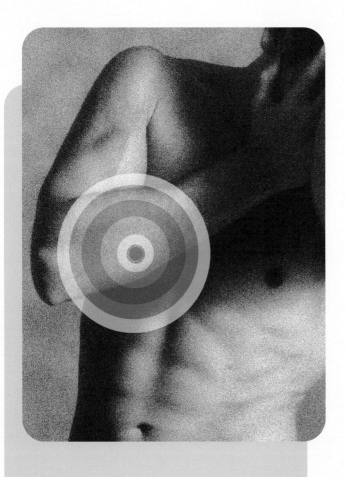

Inflammation
Magnets to use: one 2000 gauss

Inflammation is the body's natural response to any invasion by a toxic agent. Examples include wasp stings, nettle rash, rashes, burns, or scalds. The inflammation is a sign that there is more blood at the wound site than under normal conditions. The white cells in this blood protect us from such invasions and their presence is an indispensable part of the healing process.

Magnets reduce inflammation by increasing the flow of blood away from the wound site. Apply the magnet directly to the affected area, held in place with a bandage. Acute pain should subside almost immediately, but leave the magnet on overnight to reduce the inflammation.

Headaches
Magnets to use: one 200–700 gauss

Many headaches will be relieved by applying a magnet to the middle of the forehead, especially tension headaches or migraines which can be caused by constriction in the blood vessels in the head. Keep the magnet in place for 10–15 minutes, attached to a hat, or just hold it on your forehead while you relax, preferably lying down.

Since headaches can arise from a large number of causes it is not possible to claim universally beneficial effects from magnets, and they are sometimes only partially successful. If after one hour the magnet has not had an effect, it is wise to discontinue the magnet treatment. On the other hand, if the magnet treatment works you can safely repeat it for up to an hour daily.

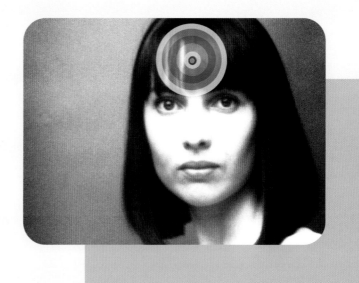

Jet lag
Magnets to use: one 2000 gauss

This condition may be caused by the rapid reorientation of the geomagnetic field in relation to the brain's own circadian rhythms. The magnet seems to act like a videotape eraser, allowing the brain to reset its clock more quickly. Place it in the centre of the forehead, either in a hat or held by hand, for the last 10 minutes of the flight.

I had a testimonial from a British woman who regularly visits relatives in Australia. After following the above instructions she had no jet lag after a flight, for the first time ever.

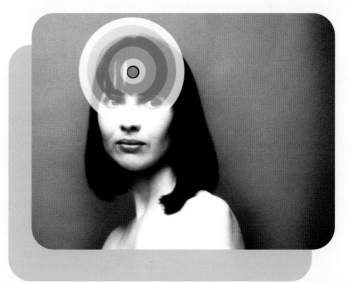

• insomnia

Some thirty million Americans and ten million British citizens now suffer from sleep disorders. Is it that they do not get physically tired, is the city air bad for them, or is it the effect of electropollution? There is much anecdotal evidence and some trial results that suggest that sleeping on a magnetic mattress improves sleep.

Magnetized mattresses

The first magnetized mattresses were manufactured in Japan and came accompanied by claims that some ten million Japanese slept on them to the benefit of their health. Since the Japanese are used to sleeping on the floor with a hard pillow, these first mattresses were often too firm for European or US taste, with some users finding that they slept worse than before. Now a wide variety of softer magnetized mattresses – or magnetized pads to put on top of normal mattresses – are available, from a range of manufacturers (see resources on page 120).

Sleeping soundly

It is a good idea to take an occasional break from the magnetic mattress, so that your body's systems do not become immune to its beneficial effects.

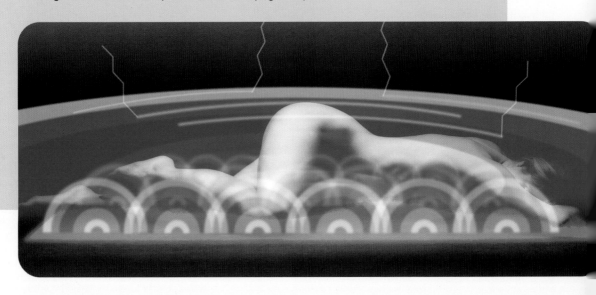

Most magnetized mattresses have around 200–300 small magnets of 750–900 gauss embedded in their foam interior, arranged with alternate north and south faces uppermost. The producers claim a wide range of benefits from sleeping on them, including improved sleep pattern, freedom from muscle pain and stiffness, and even facial rejuvenation, due to improved blood circulation.

So far I have found only one peer-reviewed study showing that magnetic mattress pads are beneficial to health (see research below). I expect that other such studies will be available soon.

Research

One joint double-blind study at three Japanese hospitals (Kaoseikai Suzuki, San-ikukai, and Tokyo Communications Hospitals; Shimodair, 1990) studied the sleep patterns of 431 people. Of these 56 slept on non-magnetized dummy mattresses, while the others had mattresses containing 104 magnets of 750–950 gauss. After six months' use those with the magnetized mattresses reported a 76–95 per cent improvement in sleep. More than 50 per cent reported an improvement within three days, and this rose to 70 per cent after five days. No abnormal effects were found in the digestive, circulatory, or neuroperceptive systems after six months' use.

Research

One of the main causes of sleep disturbance in otherwise healthy individuals is the effect of electric fields in the home (see page 40). In a study by Coghill Research Laboratories we tried to evaluate the effect of the mattress' magnetic field on the electric environment of the person sleeping on it.

For several days we logged the electric field in the test area with and without the mattress. Without the mattress we saw an irregular pattern of electric field strength in the sleeping area, originating from changes in electricity use, such as switching lights and electrical appliances on and off. With the magnetic mattress in place these changes and variations were smoothed considerably.

The magnetic fields, though extremely low at a distance of 10–20cm (4–8in) from the mattress surface (in other words at user distances), clearly had an effect on the electric fields in the bedroom. The magnetic field seems to stabilize external electric fields so that they become less turbulent and so cannot interfere as much with the body's endogenous fields and cell processes.

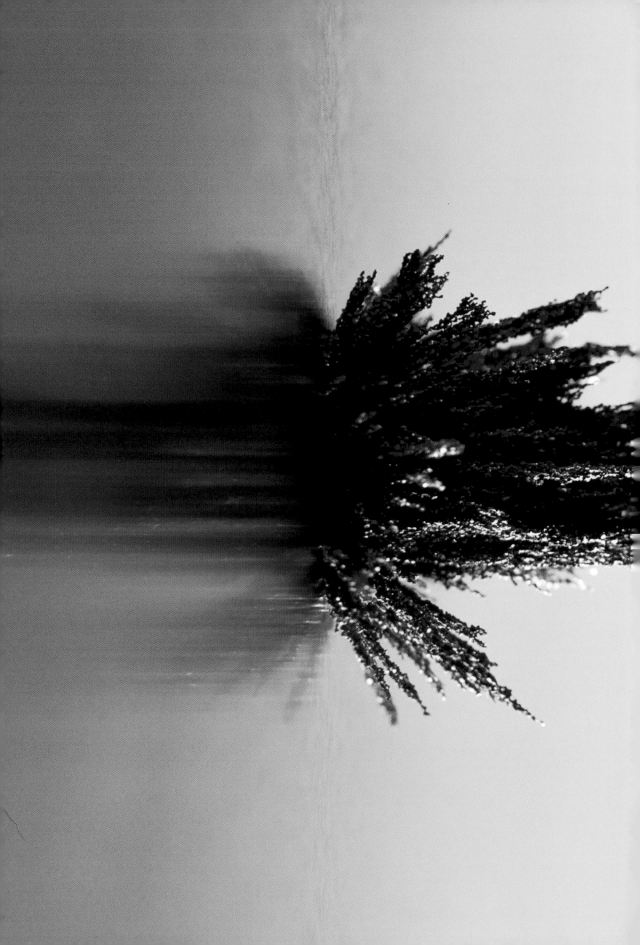

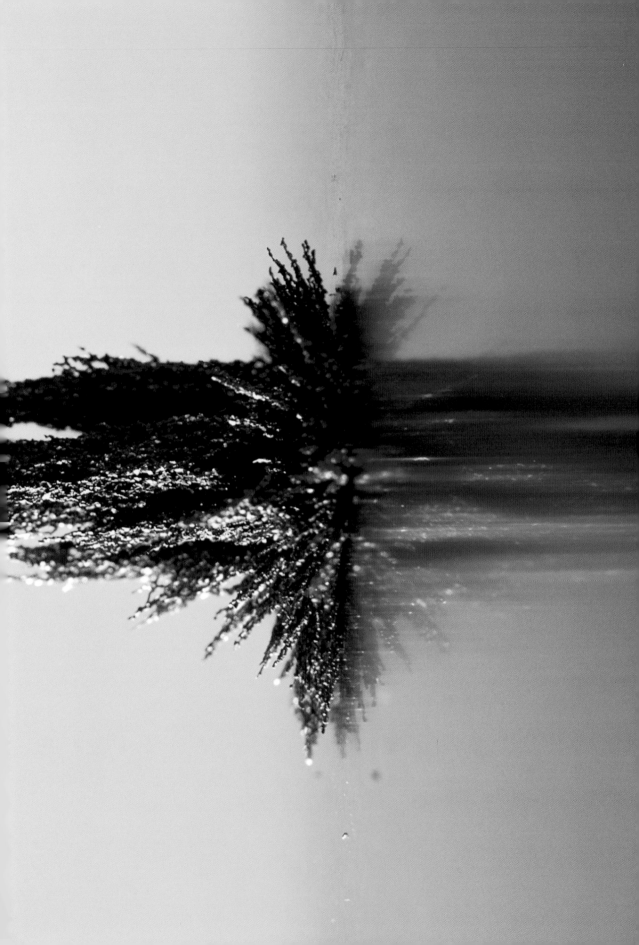

pulsating devices

Devices that mimic the body's own pulsed electric fields may have healing effects.

Many studies claiming to investigate magnetic fields have in fact investigated alternating fields, such as those emitted by electrical appliances and radio or microwave sources. The evidence seems to suggest that in general such alternating fields are harmful to the human body and its delicate endogenous electric fields (see pages 38–9).

Paradoxically, a variety of pulsating devices for healing have appeared on the market. These emit alternating current and their producers claim that they assist with problems such as sleep disturbance or lack of energy, or that they protect from other harmful radiations. At Coghill Research Laboratories we have attempted to test these devices from time to time, and there is no doubt that they do have a biological effect. Whether this effect is beneficial or not is more difficult to determine.

One problem in assessing the efficacy of these devices is that they expose the patient to a number of different parameters simultaneously: the electric component at varying frequency, the magnetic component, the varying power density of both of these, the duration of exposure, or the number of applications. The question is, which of these, or what combination, is actually doing the healing?

Another difficulty is that only one frequency has been allocated for pulsating medical devices – 27.12MHz – chosen to avoid interference with radio stations. So most studies have been able to use only that frequency.

For these reasons few pulsating devices have been cleared for medical use by the regulatory authorities – the FDA in the US and the UK Medical Devices Agency. A high level of proof of efficacy is required, since pulsating devices impart electron energy to the body, and as this builds up it must come to a point where it is harmful. As an example, cellphones are pulsating devices, and there is an increasing concern that they are causing serious long-term health effects for excessive users (see page 52).

Over the years I have received mixed reactions from patients reporting their experiences with virtually every type of pulsating device available. I can think of at least a half dozen that appeared briefly on the market and later disappeared.

Those few devices sold without practitioner supervision normally provide specific treatment instructions, and have a money-back guarantee period while you try them. In response to pressure from the UK Medical Devices Agency, the FDA in the US, and advertisement regulatory authorities seeking proof of efficacy, manufacturers are commissioning peer-reviewed scientific studies to investigate their claims.

Affecting the brain's electrical activity

Electroencephalograms (EEGs) measure the electrical activity of the brain. First discovered in 1929, the function of these EEG rhythms is still largely unknown. We know that they change during illness, and that they are individual to each of us, like DNA. One theory is that the brain's EEG records are a crude reflection of a much more sophisticated signalling system, which the brain uses to order and control cell functions.

Stephen Walpole, a British electrical engineer, became interested in EEGs after a car accident left him with severe migraine attacks. From studying EEG measurements taken from a large number of different people, he deduced that migraine sufferers were lacking certain frequencies in their EEG patterns. These missing frequencies varied between individuals. This led him to suspect that migraines, and possibly other ailments such as chronic fatigue syndrome, arise from the loss of EEG frequencies. He invented a device, the Empulse, that could identify the missing frequencies and emit them artificially, and when he found it substantially reduced his own migraines he started producing it commercially. Controversy surrounds his device, but one study has found it effective for some patients (see left).

Pages 102–7 describe research and possible treatments for a variety of conditions. Since pulsating devices vary from manufacturer to manufacturer, it is not possible to give a general treatment plan. Follow the manufacturer's instructions, or consult a magnet therapist.

Case study

A clinical trial of the Empulse device technique was published by Sophie Young in the *Journal of Alternative and Complementary Medicine* in 1988. She found that one third of a group of 54 migraine sufferers stopped having migraine attacks altogether after a three-month trial, as long as they continued wearing the device. After adjustments to the frequencies being emitted, even the remaining patients stopped having migraine attacks.

- migraine
- depression

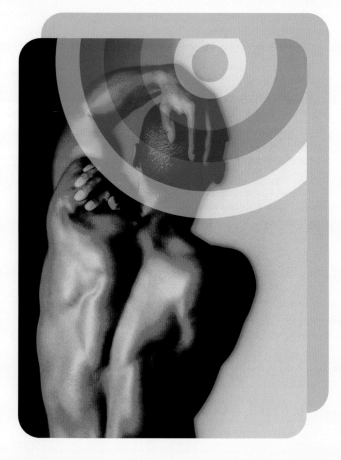

Migraine

EmWave (Empulse) devices (see page 101) first measure the patient's EEG rhythms and can then be programmed to pulse out the brain's missing frequencies, which some sufferers find alleviates migraine. Before you can use the device an EmWave practitioner uses a scanning headset to establish which brain frequencies are lacking. The device is then programmed to emit these, and is worn around the neck at all times.

Cheaper devices are available that pulse in a fixed range of frequencies, but these are not tailored to the individual and so may not be as effective in all cases.

Depression

The front cover of *New Scientist* in August 1995 declared that "Happiness is a magnet!". Inside, it explained that Mark George and co-researchers at Washington's National Institute of Health had found that applying very strong pulsating magnetic fields to the left pre-frontal cortex for 20 minutes every other day relieved depressive illness in a 40-year-old woman who had attempted suicide, had been admitted to hospital five times, and had a long list of failed medication. The pre-frontal cortex is an area of the brain often found to be underactive in depressed patients.

The technique they used, called transcranial magnetic stimulation (TMS), was pioneered in London's Institute of Neurology by Pat Merton and John Rothwell in the 1990s. It was first used to diagnose strokes, tumors, and other brain impairments, and then found applications in Parkinson's disease. The magnetic activity revives neural activity in a part of the brain often numbed in people with chronic depression, but the technique is still in an experimental stage.

Seasonal Affective Disorder

The cause of this winter depression is disturbed levels of melatonin – the hormone secreted by the pineal gland that helps regulate the body clock. Melatonin levels depend on light and darkness: high levels produced at night (in the dark) make us feel sleepy.

Melatonin production can also be affected by artificial magnetic fields, and some scientists have suggested that cyclical daily and annual changes in the geomagnetic field may be important in adjusting melatonin rhythms.

However the strongest effect on the pineal gland and melatonin production is due to bright light entering the eye. A treatment that has shown promising results is for the depressed patient to sit in front of a light box for an hour or so first thing in the morning. To regulate melatonin production effectively the light must be about 2500 lux – much brighter than indoor lighting levels, which tend to be less than 1000 lux.

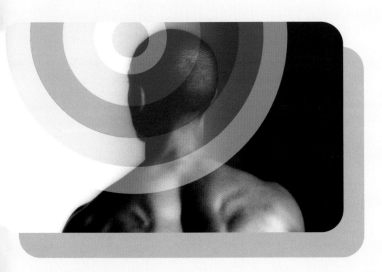

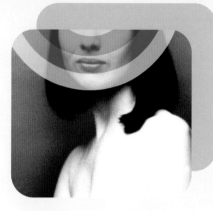

- cystitis
- sinusitis
- insomnia

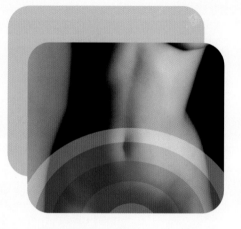

Sinusitis

In a controlled trial carried out in 1988 on 99 children with sinusitis, Czech researcher Jiri Jerabek used a Russian device (JLM1) to apply a 25Hz pulsed field of around 30 gauss to the sinuses for 20 minutes each day. In 62 of the 72 children treated the sinusitis cleared, compared with only four of the 17 children in the control group.

The most effective treatment was to use the pulsed magnetic therapy (PMT) in conjunction with antibiotics which had previously been ineffective used on their own. Almost as effective was treatment with PMT combined with decongestant nasal drops. The PMT was only used as a last resort after other attempts with the drops and antibiotics alone, as well as other treatments, had failed.

Cystitis

The Russians have pioneered the use of magnetic fields to alleviate the pain of cystitis. In a 1971 study of 188 women with adnexitis, a related condition causing inflammation of the ovaries, Komendryan used a pulsed 25 gauss field at 50Hz, for five minutes (20 applications). The patients reported almost immediate relief and palpation pains ceased. Another research group (Vasilchenko, Berlin et al) in 1976 used a slightly longer exposure period – up to 15 minutes – in the lower back and abdomen areas on 53 women with fallopian tube inflammation. All the patients reported pain relief after the third or fourth exposure.

Insomnia

Sleep disturbance is so common these days it has become almost endemic. Not surprisingly a number of instruments have appeared claiming to treat insomnia effectively, and most of these rely on pulsed magnetic fields. Over the years several products have been marketed, often with only limited success before their producers went out of business. Perhaps they did not take off in sales terms because there are few peer-reviewed studies available to support their claims.

Electromagnetic therapy devices for sleep induction typically pulse at pre-selected rates chosen by the user. The manufacturers claim that they mimic the brain's slow rhythms observed during sleep. These slow pulses, usually around 4–6Hz, have a calming and sleep inducing effect. They are used overnight, either placed under the pillow or within 1m (3ft) of the body. The devices are capable of delivering a wide range of frequencies and field strengths and all have their own instructions for use, plus a list of contraindications.

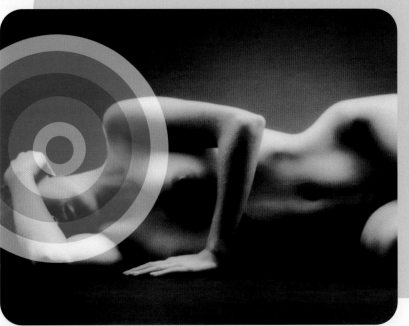

biomagnetic acupuncture

Acupuncture techniques are now commonly used in the west to treat a wide variety of conditions.

The theory of traditional Chinese medicine is set out in a treatise dating from 200BC, the Nei Ching or *The Yellow Emperor's Classic of Internal Medicine*. Life energy or chi flows through the body along pathways called meridians. In health this flow is smooth and harmonious, but in disease the flow may be unbalanced or even blocked. The acupuncture points on the meridians are points where the flow of chi can be manipulated and rebalanced to promote health, either using needles (acupuncture), pressure (acupressure), or burning herbs (moxibustion).

Electro-acupuncture is a more modern innovation, where a weak electric current is applied to the acupuncture needles. Most acupuncture equipment suppliers offer electro-acupuncture instruments, but they should only be used by trained acupuncture practitioners. Another recent development is to combine magnet therapy with acupuncture, applying magnets instead of needles to the acupuncture points.

The electrical qualities of meridians

One of the first scientists to explore acupuncture from an electromagnetic viewpoint was Dr Robert Becker, working in Albany, New York, in the early 1970s. He was interested in the use of acupuncture in Chinese hospitals for pain relief during and after surgical operations, and suggested that the acupuncture meridians were electrical conductors carrying signals to the brain, including injury messages. If this were so, blocking these pathways with acupuncture needles might prevent the pain message reaching the brain.

With a small grant from the US National Institute of Health, Becker and his colleague Dr Maria Reichmanis, a biophysicist, mapped out the electrical conductivity of the skin around the meridians. To their astonishment they found the acupuncture points were positively charged compared with their environs, and were surrounded by an electric field. They also found a fifteen minute rhythm in the current strength on the skin surface at the acupuncture points, with a decreasing field gradient as the probe moved away from the points, and published four papers on the topic.

With this understanding of acupuncture points' electrical nature, it is clear that inserting a needle at such a point will affect the flow of electric current. Applying static magnets to the acupuncture points will influence the flow of electric current in a similar manner, by diverting the electron pathway (see left).

Treating stress with electro-acupuncture

Dr Saul Liss, a consultant at MEDIConsultants Inc of Paterson, New Jersey, has researched cranial and acupuncture sites in collaboration with Norman Shealy of the Shealy Institute, Springfield, Missouri. At the 10th International Montreux Congress on Stress in 1999 he reported a study on neurotensin, a powerful neurochemical originating in the brain's hypothalamus. Electro-acupuncture was applied to thirteen different acupuncture points five days a week for five minutes each time, and the level of neurotensin measured before and after. They found that the neurotensin levels were raised significantly by the electro-acupuncture treatment, and observed a marked reduction in stress and depression in the subjects. The pioneering work of Luo, Meng and colleagues in Japan in 1998 also demonstrated that in treating depressive disorders, electro-acupuncture was just as effective as treatment with the drug amitryptiline.

Developing treatments

Various devices on the market apply therapeutic alternating electromagnetic frequencies to acupuncture points to treat conditions as diverse as headaches, migraine, muscular, arthritic and rheumatic pains, and amputation pain. A number of studies have shown that treatment with magnets on acupuncture points gives beneficial results.

This whole field is so new that treatments are still being developed and it is important to work with a qualified acupuncturist. Once you have been instructed in the technique, you may well be able to treat yourself at home.

Magnetic clamping

A flow of electric current is simply a flow of electrons, and a magnetic field will make the electrons all spin in one direction. Dr Robert Becker found that a strong enough magnetic field at right angles to an acupuncture "current" in an animal magnetically clamped it, stopping the flow. He used frogs and salamanders, placed between the poles of a magnet so that the top-to-tail current observed in their bodies was at right angles to the magnetic field. The animals were anesthetized by the magnetic field, and their EEG records showed no difference to those produced under drug-induced anesthetic.

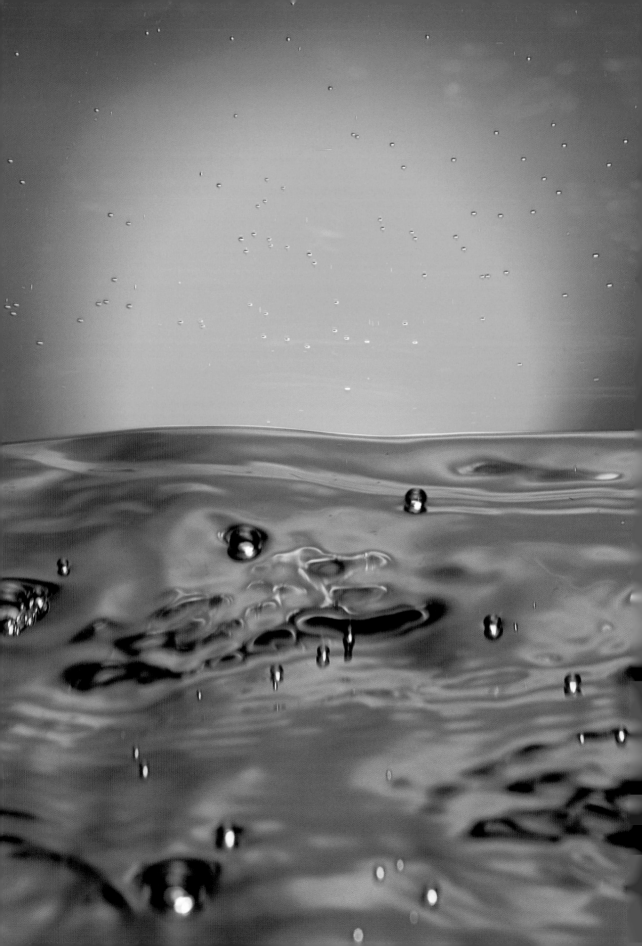

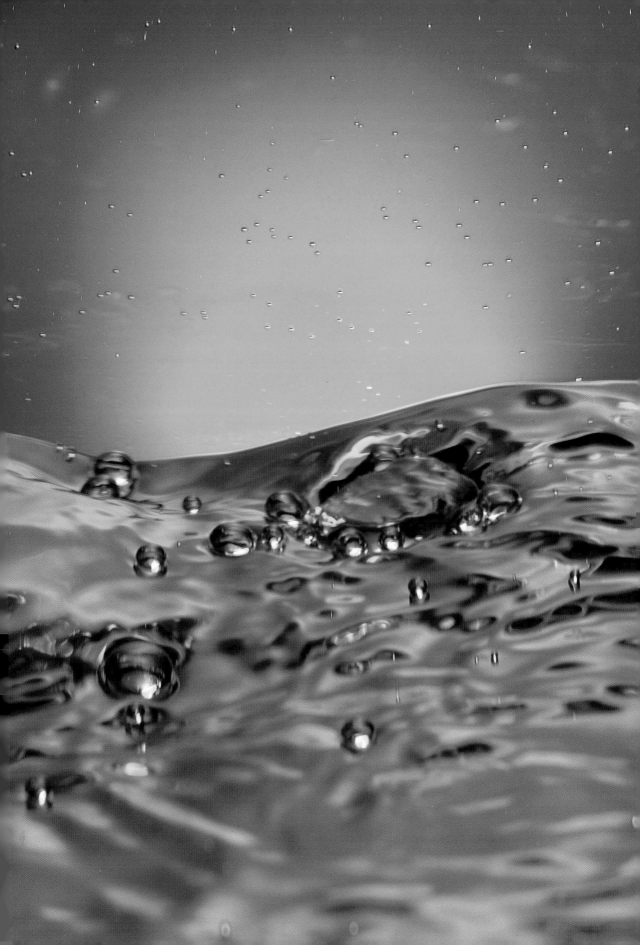

magnetized water

Drinking magnetized water daily takes the power of magnets inside your body.

Use de-ionized water if possible (the type used to top up car batteries), but do not use distilled water. You can also achieve good results with tap water. The water should be in a clean glass, ceramic, or stainless steel container. You can treat up to one litre (two pints) at a time following these instructions.

Use as powerful a magnet as you can, up to a maximum of 10,000 gauss.

Method

Place two magnets on the container, one on either side, with opposite poles facing inward. You will know that you have the opposite poles, as they will attract each other. Attach the magnets with tape. Alternatively simply place a magnet under the container of water.

Expose the water for a minimum of 30 minutes – preferably leave overnight.

It is possible to buy patented magnetic mugs that work by the same principles to magnetize water in 30 minutes (see resources on page 120).

Once the magnets are removed the magnetized water will stay effective only if it is protected from artificial magnetic fields from domestic sources such as nearby electrical appliances. Therefore it is best to drink it when it is freshly prepared, for example first thing in the morning if exposed overnight.

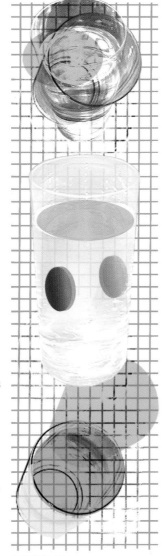

Drink 300–500ml (½ pint) daily. Magnetized water is safe for anyone of any age and can be taken on its own or with fruit juices or other drinks. Some claim it improves the taste of juices, or even Scotch whisky. Boiling or heating will destroy the effects of the magnet, so drink the water cold.

Do not use magnetized water to take prescribed drugs or other medication, since there is evidence that magnets increase the take-up of medication in the body and you could be affected more than the recommended dose expects (see page 82).

Case study

Dick Wicks of Glenhuntly, Victoria, suffered chronic pain from gout for 20 years. On the advice of a Chinese specialist from Beijing he started drinking magnetized water daily. Since the first day of this treatment he has not had another gout attack, and after two years blood tests showed that his uric acid level (high in gout sufferers) had returned to normal.

Wicks now runs a long-established and flourishing magnetic therapy business in Australia and has developed magnetic drinking mugs, known as Wicks mugs, to magnetize water, as well as a wide range of other magnet products.

Case study

Dan Watt, Cecilia Rosenfelder, and their colleagues at George Mason University, Virginia investigated the use of magnetized water to prevent the build-up of plaque on teeth. It is well established that magnets can reduce "furring" in plumbing pipework (see page 35). These researchers had the bright idea that the same principle could be applied to oral hygiene.

They set up a double-blind trial with 64 Hydrofloss oral irrigation devices, designed to include a magnetizing component. Unknown to those taking part in the trial, this magnetizing component was removed from about half the devices. The irrigation devices were then supplied to 54 patients with severe plaque build-up.

The results showed that the formation of plaque and calculus was greatly reduced in the patients using the irrigator with magnetizing device, compared with the controls.

Health benefits from magnetized water

Although there has been little research into the health benefits of drinking magnetized water, anecdotal evidence shows that it has important benefits for general wellbeing, and also in treating some common conditions and ailments.

Exposing water to a magnetic field arranges the water molecules in a more precise order. When this water is drunk, it is believed that the ordering of the molecules makes it easier for the body's cells to ingest nutrients through the body tissues' water-based bathing fluids, and to expel waste products more efficiently. Thus the cells have more energy for the body to use where it is needed.

Increased vitality	As the body's cells seem to operate more efficiently, general vitality increases after a month or so of drinking magnetized water daily.
Relief from back pain	More efficient cell function gives more energy to tired muscles so they support the skeleton better and back pain disappears.
Improved circulation	The heart beats more easily, and the blood flows through veins and arteries more efficiently, so blood pressure problems normalize.
Oral hygiene	Magnetized water reduces plaque build-up – see case study, left.
Intestinal problems	Gastrointestinal problems, such as constipation and diarrhea, tend to normalize.

magnets' influence on water

Many claims have been made for the health benefits of magnetized water. But how does it work?

Natural fresh spring water is slightly magnetized by the Earth's magnetic field and is electrically neutral. In contrast the water that comes into our homes through pipes suffers electron "damage" as friction between the water and the pipes knocks off electrons (see page 32) and is exposed to stray alternating electric fields. It also has chemicals added to it, such as chlorine for purification, and fluoride in some areas. We are not drinking a healthy fluid! So it is no wonder that so many people have turned to natural bottled spring water.

For over ten years the Japanese have used magnetized water to help control high blood pressure and diabetes. In his book *Magnet Therapy,* Dr Paul Rosch argues that when water moves through a magnetic field the hydrogen ions and dissolved minerals within it become charged and help form the water molecules into clusters. This both improves the water's taste and makes it softer. Other claims made for magnetized water are that it keeps the blood free of impurities, reduces excess cholesterol, dissolves kidney stones, and preserves general health.

Biological effects of magnetized water

How could magnetic fields influence water enough to make it therapeutic? There are a number of speculations and hypotheses, but one thing is certain: water can store electrical energy, and later re-emit it. The pattern of this energy can be adverse or beneficial to our own natural fields. As we saw in. chapter two, alternating electric fields generally have harmful effects on living organisms. So it is important that any electric fields in drinking water should be compatible with the body's endogenous electric fields.

Professor Emilio del Giudice, from the University of Milan, has advanced the concept of super-radiance to explain how

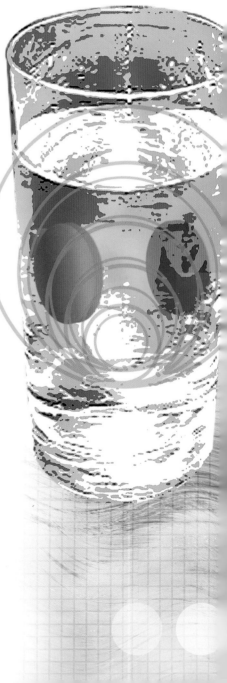

magnetized water might have a superior biological effect to normal water. In normal water the water molecules are bound together in a fairly random manner, whereas in magnetized water the molecules line up within the magnetic field. This more ordered water structure can be used more efficiently by the body's cells in ingestion of nutrients and excretion of waste products. So by magnetizing water we are preparing it for the body.

Mikhail Zhadin and Vadim Novikov are physicists from the Institute of Cell Biophysics at Pushchino, Moscow Region. Working with Frank Barnes, an electrical engineer from Colorado University, in 1998 they reported an unusual experiment. Water had various amino acids added to it and was then exposed to specific ELF frequencies and a static magnetic field simultaneously. When the frequency was tuned to resonate the amino acid (a frequency know as ion cyclotron resonance) the flow of electric current through the water suddenly increased. Without the static magnetic field the experiment did not work.

The frequency required to accelerate the conductivity depended entirely on the strength of the magnetic field. This suggests that applying a static magnetic field can alter the conductivity of water, thereby allow signalling processes to improve. If magnetized water can carry its memory of the fields it has previously been exposed to into the body, the same effect may occur at a cellular level.

Case study

At the Banaras Hindu University, India, a group headed by KK and Subas Rai reported an experiment in the journal, *Electro- and magneto biology* in 1998. They assessed the effectiveness of an insecticide, endosulfan, in killing mustard aphids. Some of the insecticide was mixed with water pre-treated by exposure to a 3000 gauss magnetic field, and some with normal water. The pre-treated insecticide solutions produced more statistically significant killing effects than any of the controls. It seems that the magnetized water made the insecticide more efficient.

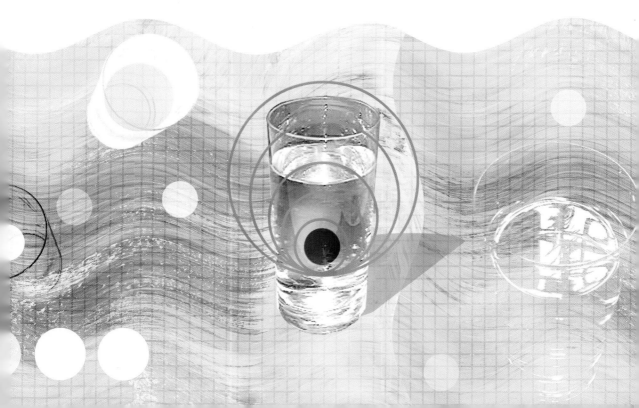

treating plants

Techniques for applying electricity and magnetism to plants have a long history.

In eighteenth century France, Abbé Jean Antoine Nollet, physics tutor to the Dauphin, believed that "electroculture" made plants grow faster. His treatise, published in 1754, described how he used metal wires to bring atmospheric electricity to the soil of plants in metallic pots, following his observations that plant growth increased where lightning struck. Nollet claimed that these treated plants grew faster than others.

In 1770 one Professor Gardini stretched electrified wires above his garden in Torino hoping to improve his crops. But the prize went to another cleric, Abbé Bertholon, who persuaded his gardener to water plants with an electrified watering can, producing lettuces of gigantic size. Bertholon's *De L'électricité des Végetaux* (On the electricity of vegetation) was the first full-scale treatise on electroculture. Bertholon went on to invent an "electrovegetometer" which collected atmospheric electricity with an antenna, and fed it via a conductor to plants growing in a field.

More recently, in 1975, GH Sidaway described some early experiments in electroculture in the *Journal of Electrostatics*. He included the technique of "artficial overhead discharge" pioneered in 1885 by Professor Lemstrom, of the University of Helsingfors, who was intrigued by the rapid plant growth at high latitudes during the short summers. Lemstrom concluded that the faster growth was because of the electric environment, and his practical studies confirmed this, published in a 1902 book *Elektrocultur*.

In the early twentieth century the UK Ministry of Agriculture carried out extensive tests to investigate whether crop yields could be improved by applying electric current. The trials were apparently successful but the results were not released and the project was mysteriously abandoned. Nevertheless the

Case study
Alexis Zrimec from Ljubljana's Bion laboratory, Slovenia reported in 1998 that watering seedlings with magnetized water improves their germination rate. He also found that seedling growth could be impaired by using water that had been exposed to alternating electric fields.

Paramagnetic antennae
Philip Callahan is an American agricultural scientist who has in the past worked with the US Department of Agriculture and as Professor of Entomology at Gainsville's University of Florida. He believes that the ancient round towers in Ireland are antennae tuned to receive atmospheric radiations in the infra red frequency range from outer space, and disseminate magnetic energy, channelling it to help plant growth. The limestone, basalt, and sandstone used to build these towers are all paramagnetic. This means that they are susceptible to magnetic fields and can keep them stored within them.

idea lingered on. This approach is described in detail in two fascinating books: *The Secret Life of Plants* and *The Secrets of the Soil*, by Christopher Bird and Peter Tompkins.

There are also reports that exposure to electric fields and radiation can damage plants. Several studies carried out in Latvia in 1996, into the effects of high intensity radio waves from a surveillance system, reported genetic damage to pine cones, and duckweed that grew upside down in the path of the beam. Hearsay reports during the cold war claimed that pine forests close to East German border radar locations were devastated by the microwaves. Until we understand better the mechanisms at work it would be wise not to apply electric currents directly to your pet houseplants, or to stand them near sources of electric fields such as televisions and other electrical appliances (see chapter two).

Using magnetic fields

Magnetism has also been used to treat plants, by watering with magnetized water or by applying magnetic fields to the plant. In 1960 LJ Audus, a botany professor at London's Bedford College, while researching the effects of gravity on plants stumbled on the discovery that their roots are sensitive to magnetic fields. His pioneering paper in the journal *Nature* "Magnetotropism, a new plant growth response" quickly brought others into the field, including Krylov and Tarakanova who demonstrated that tomato plants ripen faster near the south pole of a magnet.

Some remarkable new developments in magnetic field applications are now reaching the marketplace. Abe Liboff and colleagues at Oakland University have developed a small "black box" that applies specific magnetic fields to valuable indoor plants, such as orchids. Orchids take several years to germinate, with sterile conditions essential, and some flower only after twelve years, so speeding up the process can be important commercially.

The machinery inside the black box senses the level of the Earth's magnetic field and then emits an artificial magnetic field frequency to augment it, creating the frequency required for resonance of the plant's nutrient ions. When this occurs the plant's nutrient intake is increased and trials have shown that growth is significantly accelerated. A miniaturized device is now patented for commercial sale.

Magnetized water for plants

In the absence of more research in this promising field I cannot guarantee that using magnetized water will improve the growth of your plants, but given the health benefits it has for humans, it seems to be worth experimenting with it.

Follow the instructions for magnetizing water on page 110, using rainwater rather than tap water, and use it to water plants indoors or in the greenhouse. Seedlings in particular should benefit (see case study left).

To magnetize larger quantities of water place a coated neodymium magnet in a rainwater butt. Use as strong a magnet as possible, up to 10,000 gauss. In addition, ensure that the water butt is not sited near electricity installations such as power lines, substations, or mains electricity meters, so that it is not exposed to alternating electric fields.

For watering plants in the garden, fix magnets around a hosepipe. The type that you can buy to protect plumbing from limescale build-up will do. As well as magnetizing the water, the magnets will keep the nutrient ions needed by plants (calcium, potassium, etc) in solution and therefore more accessible to them.

treating animals

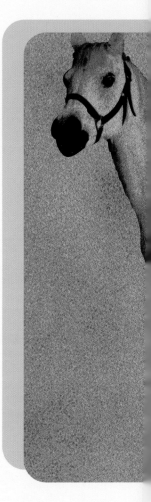

Magnet therapy's success in treating animals is now widely accepted.

Many people have been encouraged to try using magnets for their own ailments after seeing the beneficial effects on their pets. The applications are still being discovered, but do not be afraid to try when there seems no other possibility, or consult a magnet therapist. You will know within a few days if an improvement has occurred.

Always consult your veterinary surgeon before trying to treat any animal, since you may do more harm than good if you have not diagnosed the problem correctly.

• horses

Treating horses with magnets is now fairly mainstream, particularly for racehorses, where a sprain or joint problem can mean the loss of prize money or stud fees. Specialist equestrian magnet firms sell a wide variety of products, but you can achieve results more cheaply using standard neodymium magnets attached with bandages. Remember that horses roll and are very active, so keep the horse in the stable overnight for the treatment, so it will be easier for you to find the magnet if it becomes dislodged.

Worms
Magnets to use: 4000 gauss

Horses need to be wormed at least every three months, and the normal treatment with piperazine powders can be very expensive. Also, the worm treatment used has to be changed every year or so to avoid intestinal problems.

To clear worms, apply the magnets on the girth of the horse's rug, holding them in place with a coin on the other side, and leave them on overnight for several weeks.

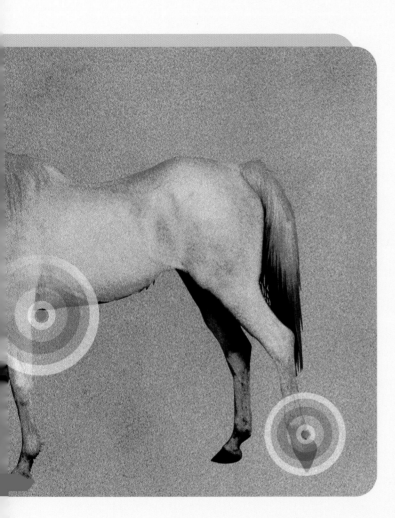

Laminitis
Magnets to use: 1000 gauss

In this common hoof problem, sometimes caused by grazing in long wet grass, blood flow to the hoof is restricted, impoverishing its oxygen supply. The hoof then becomes soft, spongy, and painful.

The magnets should be applied to the back of the foot just above the hoof. They can be held in place with a normal travelling shoe or bandage, or a sock manufactured with the magnets in place, available from equine magnet suppliers (see resources on page 120). Leave the magnets on for part of each day or overnight, and continue the treatment until the condition is cured.

Case study
In a published study on laminitis funded by Norfield, an equine magnet distributor, researchers used a technique called scintigraphy to measure the effectiveness of static magnets applied in a hoof boot. Scintigraphy involves injecting a radiolabelled substance into the bloodstream and X-raying the hoof to see where the radioactive injection has gone. Horses exposed to 1000 gauss static magnets for some weeks showed significant improvements in blood circulation in their treated hooves compared with untreated controls.

Sprains
Magnets to use: 4000 gauss

Apply the magnet to the affected joint with a bandage or leg protector overnight, until the sprain is cured.

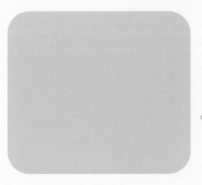

• cats and dogs

The disorders common in household pets mirror our own common ailments, and largely for the same reasons: lack of exercise and a sedentary lifestyle leading to arthritic and circulatory conditions. Pets can also suffer adverse effects from exposure to electric fields, just as we do. How often have you noticed that the place you select for the dog or cat basket is unacceptable to the pet, who goes off to sleep somewhere else?

Cats, unlike dogs, seem to prefer a slightly "electric" place, but too strong a field will be harmful. Avoid making your pet's sleeping area next to an electrical appliance, such as an electric room heater, although it seems warm and cosy.

Applying magnets to animals is tricky, and they can become skilful at dislodging them unless securely fixed. The easiest way is to make or buy a cloth jacket to fit your pet, that fastens securely underneath. Hold the magnets in place in the jacket with a coin on the other side of the fabric.

Arthritis
Magnets to use: 750 gauss

Apply the magnets overnight, on the affected area, for up to one week. Usually there will be a noticeable improvement in this time. If you cannot apply the magnets to the area affected, a magnet on the collar overnight can have good results.

Case study
My collie dog suffered from arthritic pain, so I tried attaching a magnet to her collar overnight. The morning after her first treatment I was horrified to find her with her neck bent at an odd angle. Panic – until I realized that the magnet had attached itself to a metal support just by the door! A salutary lesson: when wearing a powerful magnet you may have the same sort of encounter with the kitchen refrigerator.

However, the arthritis treatment was effective. The dog was noticeably more mobile within a week, judged by how she jumped up at the word "walkies" – a crude but effective test.

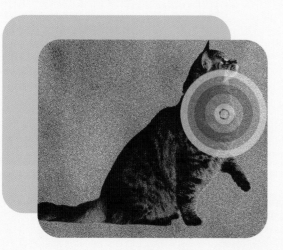

Worms
Magnet to use: four 750 gauss

Worms are commonly treated with piperazine worming powders, and most pets have to be wormed every three to six months, which can be quite expensive. Place four magnets on the front of the abdomen for the first night, then shift them to the middle of the abdomen for the second night, and to the lower abdomen for the third. The treatment may cause slight diarrhea. For optimum results give the cat or dog magnetized drinking water too.

Bone fractures
Sometimes fractures will not heal successfully, particularly in pregnancy when essential supplies of calcium are being diverted into the fetus. A pulsating electromagnetic field which mimics the bone's own piezoelectric action can help the healing process. Several firms manufacture devices for this type of treatment, but it should always be supervised by your veterinary surgeon.

Case study
A friend's lurcher bitch had been kicked by a horse while pregnant, and the bone would not heal. I provided a pulsating device with a frequency of 50Hz which was bandaged to the leg for around 30 minutes each day. The vet also provided additional calcium supplements. The fracture eventually healed successfully.

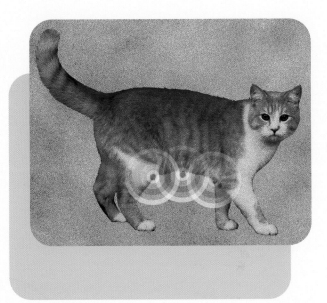

resources
bibliography

Baker, Douglas
Biomagnetism
De la Warr Laboratories, 1972

Bansal, Dr H L
Magnetotherapy Self Help Book
B Jain Publishers, New Delhi, India, 1989

Bansal, Dr H L
Magnetic Cure for Common Diseases
Vision Books, 1984

Barnothy, Madeleine
Biological Effects of Magnetic Fields
Plenum Press Inc, New York, 1964

Bengali, Neville S
Magnet Therapy Theory and Practice
B Jain Publishers, New Delhi, India, 1995

Berthon, Simon; Robinson, Andrew
The Shape of the World
Guild Publishing, 1991

Burke, Abbot G
Magnetic Therapy: healing in your hands
Devorss & Co, 1987

Callahan, P
Ancient mysteries, modern visions: the
magnetic life of agriculture
Acres, USA, Kansas City, MO, 1984

Coghill, Roger (editor)
Proceedings of 1st World Congress in
Magnetotherapy
Coghill Research Laboratories, 1997

Coghill, Roger
Something in the Air
Coghill Research Laboratories, 1998

Collinson, Gayel
Magnets Restore Health
Desk Top Publishing
Tauranga, New Zealand, 1994

Davis, Albert Roy
The Magnetic Blueprint of Life
Acres USA, Kansas City MO, 1979
Available from:
ARD Research Laboratory
520 Magnolia Avenue

Green Cove Springs
Florida 32043, USA
Tel: 001 904 264 8564

Davis, Albert Roy; Rawls, Walter C
The Magnetic Effect
Acres USA, Kansas City MO, 1975;
available as above

Davis, Albert Roy; Rawls, Walter C
Magnetism and its effects on the living
system
Acres USA, Kansas City MO, 1976;
available as above

Downing, Dr Damien
Daylight Robbery: the importance of
sunlight to health
Arrow Books Ltd, 1988

Gilbert, William
De Magnete
Dover Publications, 1991

Gordon, Rolf
Are you sleeping in a safe place?
Dulwich Health, 130 Gipsy Hill, London
SE19 1PL, 1988

Hannemann, Prof Holger
Magnet Therapy: balancing your body's
energy flow for self-healing
Sterling Publishing Company, 1990

Jerabek, Jiri; Pawluk, William
Magnetic Therapy in Eastern Europe:
a review of 30 years of research
William Pawluk, 1998

Morris, Noel C
The Book of Magnetic Healing and
Treatments
Redwing Book Co, Brookline, MA 02136

Null, Gary
Healing with Magnets
Constable Robinson, 1998

Payne, Buryl
The Body Magnetic
Psychophysics, 1992

Philpott, William H; Taplin, Sharon
Biomagnetic Handbook: a guide to medical
magnets
Enviro-Tech Products, 1990
Reproduced in the UK by Health Vitalics,
Great Bookham, Surrey

Rinker, Fred
The Invisible Force: traditional magnetic
therapy
Mass Market Pubs, 1997
Available from: Mason Service Publishing
CP27106, London, Ontario, Canada
N5X 3X5
Tel: 001 519 660 0491

Rosch, Paul; Lawrence, Ron; Plowden,
Judith
Magnet Therapy: the pain cure alternative
Prima Health Publishing, California, 1998

Santwani, Dr M T
The Art of Magnetic Healing
B Jain Publishers, New Delhi, India, 1986

Schul, Bill D
The Magnetic Connection
Insights Productions, Winfield, KS67156

Smyth, Angela; Thompson, Chris
Seasonal Affective Disorder: who gets it,
what causes it, how to cure it
Thorsons, 1992

Walls
Magnetic Field Therapy:
balancing your energy field
New Leaf Distribution Company, 1993

Washnis, George J; Hricak, Richard Z
Discovery of Magnetic Health
Nova Publishing Corp, Rockville,
Massachussetts, 1993

Whitaker, Julian; Adderly, Brenda
The Pain Relief Breakthrough: the power
of magnets
Little, Brown and Co, 1998

scientific references

AKOYUNOGLOU, G
Effect of a magnetic field on carboxydismutase.
Nature 1964, 202: 452–454

ARYSHENSKAYA, A M; OSIPOV, V V et al
The clinical use of magnetic fields.
Ishevsk.1977, pp64–65

AUDUS, L J
Magnetotropism: a new plant-growth response
Nature 1960, 185: 132

BARNOTHY, M
Influence of magnetic fields upon the development of tumors in mice
Proc. 1st. Natl. Biophysics Conf. Columbus OH March 1957 p735 in (Quastler & Morowitz eds) Yale Univ. Press, New Haven 1959

BASSETT, C A L; BECKER, R O
Generation of electric potentials in bone in response to mechanical stress.
Science 1962, 137: 1063

BASSETT, C A L et al
The effect of PEMFS on cellular calcium and calcification of non-unions. In: Electrical properties of bone and cartilage: experimental effects and clinical applications (Eds. C.T. Brighton, J. Black, S.R. Pollack). Grune & Stratton, New York 1979, pp427–441

BECKER, G
Communication between termites by means of biofields and the influence of magnetic and electric fields on termites. In: Electromagnetic bioinformation, (Popp, Warnke et al, eds) Urban and Schwarzenberg, Munich, 1989, pp116–127

BECKER, R O; SELDEN, G
The body electric, Wm Morrow (Quill) Publishers, NY, 1985, pp233–236

BELLOSSI, A; SUTTER-DUB, M T et al
Effects of constant magnetic fields on rats and mice: a study of weight.
Aviat. Space Environ Med 55(8): 725–730

BENEDIKT, M
Zur Magnetotherapie. Wiener medizinische Blätter 8 (37): 1117–1121 Sept. 1885

BERGER, H
Über das Elektrenkephalogram des Menschen. First Report.
Arch. für Psychiatr. & Nervenkrankheit 1929, 87: 527–570

BLAKEMORE, R P
Magnetotactic bacteria
Science (Washington) 1975, 190: 377–379

COGHILL, R W; GALONJA-COGHILL, T
Effects of RF/MW radiations at 1.8 GHz. on human peripheral blood lymphocyte viability. October 2000, Procs. of Int. Conference, St Petersburg (in press)

COGHILL, R W; GALONJA-COGHILL, T
Protective effect of a donor's endogenous electric field on lymphocyte viability.
Electro- and magnetobiology. March 2000 (in press)

DEL GIUDICE, E; DOGLIA, S et al
Structures, correlations, and electromagnetic interactions in living matter: theory and practice. In: Biological coherence and response to external stimuli (ed. Frohlich) Springer, 1988 pp49–65

DOLK, H; SHADDICK, G, et al.
Cancer incidence near radio television transmitters in GB
Amer. J. Epidemiol. 1997, 145: 1–9

ECKERT, E
Plötzlicher und unerwarteter Tod in Kleinskindesalter und elektromagnetische Felder.
Med. Klin. 1976, 71: 1500–1505 (37)

ESPINAR, A; PIERA, V et al
Histological changes during development of the cerebellum in the chick embryo exposed to a static magnetic field. Bioelectromagnetics J. 1997, 18: 36–46

FARADAY, M
Experimental researches in electricity
Taylor and Francis, London; Dover, New York (reprint), 1855, reprinted 1965

FEWS, A P; HENSHAW, D L et al
Increased exposure to pollutant aerosols under high voltage power lines.
Int. J. Radiat. Biol 1999 75 (12): 1505–1521

FULTON, J P; COBB, S et al (4–18)
Electrical wiring configurations and childhood leukemia in Rhode Island
Amer. J. Epidemiol. 1980, 111:192

GEORGE, M S et al
Changes in mood and hormone levels after rapid rate transcranial stimulation (sTMS) of the prefrontal cortex. J. Neuropsychiatry Clin. Neurosci. 1996, 8 (2): 172–180

GERASIMOV, S
Geomagnetic fields and MS
Intl. J. Altern. Comp. Med. February 1999, pp22–25

GERASIMOV, S; COGHILL, R W
A double blind placebo-controlled study assessing healing potential for the platinum photon made garments in childhood asthma. Lviv State Medical University publication, Lviv, Ukraine, 1998

GROSS, L
Bibliography of the biological effects of static magnetic fields in: Biological effects of magnetic fields, Barnothy, M (ed) Plenum Press, NY, 1964

HANSEN, K M
Some observations with a view to possible influence of magnetism upon the human organism. Acta Med. Scand. 1938, 97: 339–364

HARKINS, T T; GRISSOM, C B
Magnetic field effects on B12 ethanolamine ammonialyase: evidence for a radical mechanism.
Science 1994, 263: 958–960

HEFFERNAN, M
Effects of variable microcurrent on EEG spectra and pain control
ISSSEEM, 1996. See also: Measurement of electromagnetic field in the healing process. Procs 9th Int. Montreux Cong. on Stress, February 1997

HEY, J S
The radio universe, Pergamon Press Oxford, 1971, pp132, 134

HOLCOMB, R R; PARKER, R A et al
Biomagnetics in the treatment of human pain, past present and future. Environ. Med 1991a 8: 24–30

HOPE-SIMPSON, R E
Relationship of Influenza pandemics to sunspot cycles (M. Kingsbourn, W. Lynn Smith eds.), Charles C. Thomas, Springfield, Illinois, 1974

HOYLE, F; WICKRAMASINGHE, N C
Sunspots and influenza
Nature 1990, 343: p304

JERABEK, J et al
Prakt. Lek. 1988, 68 (10): 389-390 and Prak. Lek. 68 (13): 516–517

KALMIJN, A J
Electroperception in sharks and rays
Nature 1966, 212: 1232–1233

KALMIJN, A J; BLAKEMORE, R P
The magnetic behaviour of mud bacteria. In: Animal migration, navigation, and homing (eds Schmidt-Koenig and Keeton). Springer Verlag Berlin, 1978, pp354–355

KIRSCHVINK, J L; KIRSCHVINK ,A K; WOODFORD, B
Human brain magnetite and squid magnetometry
Ann. Intl. Conf. of IEEE Engineering in Medicine and Biology Society 1990, 12(3): 1089–1090

KOBLUK, C N; JOHNSTON, G R et al
A scintigraphic investigation of magnetic field therapy on the equine third metacarpus.
Vet. and Comp. Orthop. and Traumatol. 1994, 7: 9–13

KOMENDRIAN, V G
Reactions of biological systems on weak magnetic fields. Moscow 1971, pp59–162

KRYLOV, A V; TARAKANOVA, G A
Magnetotropism in plants and its nature. Fiziol. Rasenii 1960, 7: 191

LAI, H; SINGH, N
Acute low intensity microwave exposure increases DNA single strand breaks in rat brain cells. Bioelectromagnetics J. 1995, 16: 207–210

LEMSTROM, S
Electricity in agriculture and horticulture, Electrician Publishing Co. London, 1904

LIBOFF, A R
Cyclotron resonance in membrane transport.
In: Chiabrera et al (eds), Interactions between electromagnetic fields and cells, Plenum Press, London, 1985

LISS, S; CLOSSON, W J
Effects of magnetic stimulation on blood biochemicals. In: Procs 9th Int. Montreux Congress on Stress, Montreux, Switzerland, Feb 1997

LISS, S; SHEALY, N, et al
Findings in enhancement-neurotensin and human growth hormone using cranial and acupuncture sites. Procs. 10th Int. Montreux Congress on Stress, Montreux, Switzerland, February 1999

MAGILL, W M et al
Recognition and treatment of depression in a family medical practice. J. Clin. Psychiatry 1983, 44: 3–6 and New Scientist 1 August, 1995

MOSLAVAC, S; MOSLAVAC, A et al
Three years' clinical application of electromagnetic therapy on 1261 patients: commonly occurring conditions and patient interruptions. Procs. 1st World Congress on Magnetotherapy, London May 1996, pp79–83 (CRL publishers, Pontypool, Wales)

MYERS, A; CARTWRIGHT, R A et al
Overhead powerlines and childhood cancer.
Proc. Intl. Conf. on Electric and Magnetic fields in medicine and biology
IEEE Conf. Pub. 1985, 257: 126–130

NAKAGAWA, K
Magnetic field deficiency syndrome and magnetic treatment.
Japan Med. J. Dec 4 1976, 2745 National Council for Radiation Protection and Measurement (NCRP) draft document. Microwave News (July/August, 1995) vol 15 (4): 1–11; 12–15

NOVIKOV, V V; ZHADIN, M N
Combined action of weak constant and variable low-frequency magnetic fields on ionic currents in aqueous solutions of amino acids. Biophysics 1994, 39(1): 41–45

OSIPOV, V V; BORSHCHAR, E L et al
Use of magnetic fields in clinical medicine. Kuybyshev 1976, 63–64

RENO, V R; NUTINI, L G
Effect of magnetic fields on tissue respiration.
Nature 1963, 196: 204–205

RUZIC, R; BERDEN, M et al
The effects of oscillating EMFs on plants, Summary report.
In: Procs. 1st Int. Cong on Effects of Electricity and Magnetism on the Natural World, Funchal, Madeira, October 1998

SALFORD, L G; BRUN, A et al
Permeability of the blood brain barrier induced by 915MHz. Electromagnetic radiation Bioelectrochem. Bioenerg. 1993, 30: 293–301

SCHUMANN, W O
Über die strahlungslosen Eigenschwingungen einer leitenden Kugel, die von einer Luftschicht und einer Ionosphärenhülle umgeben ist. Z.f. Naturforschung 1954, 7a: 149–154

SHIMODAIR, K
The therapeutic effect of the magnetized mattress pad. Obstetrics and Gynecology, Tokyo, 1990

SIDAWAY, G H
Some early experiments in electroculture
J. Electrostatics 1975, 1: 389–393

SINGH, N N; RAI, K K et al
Magnetically altered water enhances endosulfan insecticidal efficacy in mustard aphids.
Electro and Magnetobiology 1998, 17(3): 415–419

SUPRUN, L Y; KHERKEVICH, S I
Use of magnetic fields and ultrasound with therapeutic aim. Leningrad Univ. 1985, 79–82

TABLADO, L; PEREZ-SANCHES, F et al
Effects of exposure to static magnetic fields on morphology & morphometry of mouse epididymal sperm. Bioelectromagnetics J. 1998, 19(6): 377–383

VALLBONA, C; HAZLEWOOD, C F et al
Response of pain to static magnetic fields in post-polio patients: a double-blind pilot study. Arch. Phys. Med. Rehabil. 1997, 78 (11): 1200–1203

VASILCHENKO, N P; BERLIN, Y V et al
The use of magnetic fields in clinical medicine. Kuybyshev, 1976 pp27–29

WARBURG, O
On the origin of cancer cell Science 1956, 123: 309–315

WARNKE, U
Information transmission by means of electrical biofields.
Electromagnetic bio-information ed F A Popp. Schwarzenberg, 1989

WATT, D L; ROSENFELDER, C et al
The effect of oral irrigation with a magnetic water device on plaque and calculus.
J. Clin. Peridontol. 1993, 20: 314–317

WERTHEIMER, N; LEEPER, E
Electrical wiring configurations and childhood cancer.
Amer. J. Epidemiol. 1979, 109: 273–84

WILTSCHO, W; MUNRO, U et al
A magnetic pulse leads to a temporary deflection in the magnetic orientation of migratory birds. Experimentia 1994, 50: 697–700

WU, J
Further observations on the therapeutic effect of magnets and magnetised water against ascariasis in children. J. Tradit. Chinese Med. 1989, 9 (2): 111–112

YANO, A; OGURA, M et al
Effect of a modified magnetic field on the ocean migration of chum salmon, Onchorhyncus keta.
First World Congress on the Effects of Electricity and Magnetism in the Natural World, Funchal, Madeira, 1998

YOUNG, S
Pilot study concerning the effects of extremely low frequency electromagnetic energy on migraine

magnet suppliers

This section presents a list of suppliers and producers of magnets and magnetic products. Most of these give a 30–90 day trial period, during which you can return the product for a full refund if you are not satisfied.

The variety of magnet therapy products and their range of field strengths is increasingly bewildering and diverse. The right field strength for one application is not necessarily correct for another and individual products can be quite expensive. So aim to select products suitable for a range of applications.

Always find out the field strength of the magnet you are buying, so that you can assess whether you can use it to treat other conditions, as described in chapter three. Coghill Research Laboratories supplies sets of two or more magnets with spacers, so a range of strengths can be applied anywhere on the body.

Centre for Implosion Research
PO Box 38
Plymouth PL7 5YX
Tel: 01752 345 552
Fax: 01752 338 569
implosionresearch@
compuserve.com
www.implosionresearch.com
Products to counter electromagnetic radiation and enhance water quality

Coghill Research Laboratories
Lower Race
Pontypool
Gwent
NP4 5UH
Tel: 01495 763 389
Fax: 01495 769 882
enquiries@mag-lab.com
www.cogreslab.demon.co.uk
Supermagnet neodymium magnets
FieldMouse biohazard monitors, publications about electropollution and magnet therapy

Digital Health Research Ltd
Suffolk Enterprise Centre
Felaw Maltings
44 Felaw Street
Ipswich
Suffolk IP2 8SJ
Tel: 01473 407 333
Fax: 01473 407 334
info@aegis-health.com
www.aegis-health.com
AegisElectromagnetic therapy device to assist natural energy balance

D Jay Ltd
113 Pope Street
Birmingham
B1 3AG
Tel: 0121 236 2073
Fax: 0121 233 4516
info@acumed.co.uk
www.acumed.co.uk
AcumedPatch for pain relief (people and animals)

Dulwich Health
130 Gypsy Hill
London
SE19 1PL
Tel: 020 8670 5883
Fax: 020 8766 6616
www.dulwichhealth.co.uk
MagneTech

Ecoflow Ltd
21 Brunel Road
Saltash
Cornwall
PL12 6LF
Bioflow
Tel: 01752 841 661
Fax: 01752 841 044
www.ecoflow.ltd.uk
Magnetic healing products for people and animals

EmDI Ltd
Suffolk Enterprise Centre
Felaw Maltings
44 Felaw Street
Ipswich
Suffolk
IP2 8SJ
Tel: 01473 407 333
Fax: 01473 407 334
info@empulse.com
www.empulse.com
Empulse: Individually fine-tuned electromagnetic therapy device

Emsfield Magnetics
62 Clifton Vale Close
Clifton
Bristol
BS8 4PY
Tel: 0800 074 8753
Fax: 0117 958 5289
(Mobile): 07977 414 513
Magno-pulseMagnetic healthcare products for people and animals

Robert Thurston
GateNet Telecommunications Ltd
Peel House
Peel Road
Skelmersdale
Lancs
WN8 9PT
Tel: 01695 731 473
Tel: 01695 503 44
gatenet@compuserve.com
Raygard
Cellphone protection

Health Alternatives
Julia Flower
Lower Farm
St Margarets Road
Alderton
Tewkesbury
Gloucestershire
GL20 8NN
Tel: 01242 620 730
Independent distributor of Nikken products

Health Alternatives
Nancy Blinkhorn
Potter's Way
Springfield Lane
Broadway
Worcestershire
WR12 7BT
Tel: 01386 853 686
Fax: 01386 854 843
blinkhorn@compuserve.com
Independent distributor of Nikken products

HoMedics (UK) Ltd
19 Branksome Avenue
Prestwich
Manchester
M25 1AG
Tel: 0161 798 5876
Fax: 0161 798 5896
www.homedicsuk.com
Extensive range of personal wellness products

Philip Barker
Life-Energies Ltd
The Coach House
The Avenue
Odstock
Salisbury
SP5 4JA
Tel: 01725 513 129
Fax: 01722 349 468
lenergies@aol.com
www.life-energies.com
Skenar Bioenergy feedback machine for healing people and animals

Lifestyle Health Centres
The Links
73 Attimore Road
Welwyn Garden City
Herts
AL8 6LG
Tel/fax: 01707 323 868
tdalink@aol.com
www.lifestylehealthcentres.com
Ear-zyProtection device for mobile phones

Magna Jewellery
PO Box 338
Edgware
Middlesex
HA8 8HZ
Tel/fax: 020 8958 9719
Magnetic bracelets, necklaces, and pet collars

MAGNETiC
Steers farm
Pigstye Green
Willingale
Ongar
Essex
CM5 0QF
Tel: 01277 896 266
Sport, etc Wrist bands, insoles, seats, collars for pets etc

MAGNETIC THERAPY LTD
Magnet House
Worsley
Manchester
M28 2PG
Tel: 0161 793 5110
Fax: 0161 728 5055
info@magnetictherapy.co.uk
www.magnetictherapy.co.uk
Mail order catalogue containing over 150 items

Magnopulse
Cromhall Farm
Easton Piercy
Chippenham
Wilts
Tel: 01179 710 710
Fax: 01179 720 720
mailbox@magnopulse.com
www.magnopulse.com
Magnetic healthcare products
for people and animals

Microshield
59 Southbury Road
Enfield
Middlesex
EN1 1PJ
Tel: 020 8363 3333
Fax: 020 8372 3232
microshld@aol.com
www.microshield.co.uk
Cellphone protection

Mr Magnet Magnetic Products
8 Flinders Court
Boronia Heights
QLD 4124
Australia
0061 (07) 3800 1242

Nikken Inc
Irvine
California
USA
Tel: 001 949 789 2000
www.nikken.com
Founded in Japan over 21
years ago, now one of the
largest magnet distributors in
the US and worldwide

Norso Biomagnetics
Gloria Vergari & Associates
15 Cotswold View
The Hollow
Bath
BA2 1HA
Tel: 01225 314 096
Fax: 01225 316 397
norsouk@aol.com
Magnetic massage tools
and magnetic therapy wraps

NRG Marketing
12 Station Road
Kenilworth
Warwickshire
CV6 1JJ
Tel: 01926 864 200
Fax: 01926 864 222
nrg@agentbase.co.uk
www.uni-tel.co.uk
ARD Anti-radiation devices for
mobile phones

Powerwatch
2 Tower Road
Sutton
Ely
Cambs
CB6 2QA
Tel: 01353 778814
www.powerwatch.org.uk
Advice and information
helpline 0897 100 800 calls
charged at £1.50 per minute
Demand switches, cables,
meters, and meter hire, etc

institutions

American Institute of Stress
124 Park Avenue
Yonkers
NY 10703, USA
Tel: 001 914 963 1200
www.stress.org

Australian College of Magnetic Therapy
PO Box 72
Inglewood, 6052
Western Australia

The US Bioelectromagnetics Society
(BEMS)
William G Wisecup, Executive Director
W/L Associates Ltd
7519 Ridge Road
Frederick, MD 21702-3519
Tel: 001 301 663 4252
Fax: 001 301 371 8955
www.bioelectromagnetics.org

British Biomagnetic Association
The Williams Clinic
31 Marychurch Road
Torquay
Devon
TQ1 3JF
Tel: 01803 293 346
grahamgardener@biomagnetics.freeserve
.co.uk

British Complementary Medicine
Association
Kensington House
33 Imperial Square
Cheltenham
GL50 1QZ
Tel: 01242 519 911
Fax: 01242 22 77 65
info@bcma.co.uk
www.bcma.co.uk

British Institute of Magnet Therapy
Coghill Research Laboratories
Lower Race
Pontypool
Gwent
NP4 5UH
Tel: 01495 752122
BIMT@mag-lab.com

British School of Yoga
Stanhope Square
Holsworthy
Devon
EX22 6DF
Training course for magnet therapists

Council for Complementary and
Alternative Medicine
63 Jeddo Road
London
W12 98Q
Tel: 020 8735 0632

European Bioelectromagnetics Association
c/o Dr Bernard Veyret
PIOM/ENSCOB
Université de Bordeaux I
33405 Talence Cédex
France
Tel: 00 33 556 370 728

Guild of Complementary Practitioners
Liddell House
Liddell Close
Finchampstead
Berkshire
RG40 4NS
Tel: 0118 973 5757
info@gcpnet.com
www.gcpnet.com

Institute for Complementary Medicine
PO Box 194
London
SE16 1QZ
Tel: 020 7237 5165

The International Commission of
Non-Ionizing Radiation
c/o Institute of Radiation Hygiene
D-85764 Oberschleissheim
Ingolstadter Landstrassen 1
Germany

Magnetic Therapists Association of
Australia, Inc
PO Box 72
Inglewood, 6052
Western Australia

index

author's acknowledgements

I would like to dedicate this book to my beloved father.

Formative influences on me include Dr William Ross Adey, Jiri Jerabek, Imants Detlavs, Sergei Gerasimov, Alasdair Philips, Simon Best, Cyril Smith, Paul Rosch, Martin Blank, Asher Sheppard, and the Bioelectromagnetics Society community, whose annual meetings provide such stimulation. Also the folks at Vanderbilt University, Nashville Tennessee, and at St Joseph's Institute, University of Western Ontario, especially Dr Frank Prato and his colleagues there. None of them are responsible for any mistakes in this book, and their opinions do not necessarily concur with mine. I also owe a debt to Grolier Encyclopaedia for being able to dip into their concise material.

Pip Morgan, Katherine Pate, and their colleagues at Gaia deserve great commendation for turning my sometimes unfocused writing into a tighter format and getting the production out in timely fashion. We all recognized that this science is unfolding before our eyes, and we have only created a snapshot of the present, when the future is much broader.

Finally I would like to thank my wife Tamara for the great sacrifices she made so that I could concentrate on writing.

publisher's acknowledgements

The publishers would like to thank: Helena Petre and Deborah Pate for research; Maggi McCormick for advice on American terms; Anne Brabyn for checking the bibliography; Lynn Bresler for proofreading and the index, and Susanna Abbott and Emma Meysey-Thompson for last-minute proofreading.

The Coghill Supermagnet Set

This unique set of two magnets has been developed at Coghill Research Laboratories, the UK's foremost independent bioelectromagnetics laboratory and centre for The British Institute of Magnet Therapy.

Each magnet set includes an instruction leaflet explaining how to adjust the field strength of the magnet to treat your ailment effectively. The Coghill Supermagnet can be safely applied directly on to the affected area.

Each set comes with a 60 day money back guarantee.

The normal price for the Coghill Supermagnet is £32.00. Readers of this book can order from Coghill Research Laboratories for £24.00 + £2.50 p&p.

Call 01495 752122 with your credit or debit card
or send a cheque payable to EMP to
Ker Menez, Lower Race, Pontypool NP4 4UH

We do not make medical claims about our magnets

~

ALSO PUBLISHED
BY GAIA BOOKS

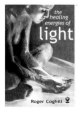

The Healing Energies of Light

Roger Coghill ISBN 1 85675 185 6 £12.99
Practical advice on bringing more light into our daily lives for better physical, emotional and spiritual wellbeing.

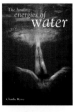

The Healing Energies of Water

Charlie Ryrie ISBN 1 85675 088 4 £12.99
Includes scientific research into vibrational energies as well as the cleansing nature of water and how it can ease many common ailments.

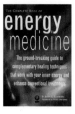

The Complete Book of Energy Medicine

Helen Dziemidko ISBN 1 85675 120 1 £14.99
A guide to over 40 complementary therapies. Work with your energy to treat ailments or to enhance conventional treatments.

To order a book or request a catalogue contact:
Gaia Books Ltd, 20 High Street, Stroud, Glos GL5 1AZ
T: 01453 752985 F: 01453 752987 E: info@gaiabooks.co.uk

visit our web site to see a complete list of our titles: www.gaiabooks.co.uk